Diet Disruption

The Weight Loss Solution
for the Chronic Serial Dieter

Jennifer Powter, MSc.

ISBN: 978-19-5-036763-4

Published by

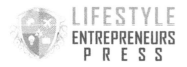
LIFESTYLE
ENTREPRENEURS
P R E S S

If you are interested in publishing through Lifestyle Entrepreneurs Press, write to:
Publishing@LifestyleEntrepreneursPress.com

Publications or foreign rights acquisition of our catalog books.
Learn More: *www.LifestyleEntrepreneursPress.com*

Printed in the USA

Advance Praise

"It's not often you come across a book on weight loss that feels so incredibly fresh and personal yet is rooted in the science and psychology of transformation. Jennifer Powter approaches this age-old struggle in such an empathetic and human way (while at the same time bringing her deeply impressive scientific expertise to bear) that you feel like you're in a one-on-one conversation with her – and that she understands what makes you tick better than you do. If you want to disrupt your habitual pattern of dieting and learn a different way to create healthy changes in your life, this book is a must-read."

—Jonathan Bailor,
New York Times Best Selling author
and founder of SANESolution

"This book is a must-read for all of the ladies out there who have been caught in the diet trap. It teaches you effective and sustainable techniques to not only lose the weight, but to also adopt a new lifestyle and learn to love your body again. I think everyone should take Jennifer's advice and ditch the diet for good!"

—Dr. Renee Wellenstein,
founder of Kaspira Eilte Health Consulting, LLC

"*Diet Disruption* is my favorite new go-to book for simple strategies that work for real women who want to enjoy their lives and not live in restriction or deprivation. The number one thing that makes weight loss hard is how complicated people make it. Jen's combination of science-based information with practical steps for optimal health and weight loss is genius. This is the book the dieting industry needs."

—Melissa Kathryn, CHHC, AADP,
HT. Int., best-selling author of Eat Right For Your
Archetype and creator of the Wholeness Podcast

"Jennifer's down-to-earth, easy-to-read book gets straight to the point about why losing weight can be challenging and how to finally keep it off for good. These simple (not easy) tactics will help thousands of people finally find a sustainable weight that's healthy for them."

—Eliza Kingsford, MA, LPC,
Amazon best-selling author of *Brain-Powered Weight Loss*

"Jen Powter puts everything on the metaphorical table in *Diet Disruption*. It is indeed, as the subtitle indicates, *the* solution for chronic dieters. By sharing her personal and clinical experience, Jen leads with empathy. Her training and references to that experience add credibility and science to back it all up. The book is filled with actionable and practical steps for letting go of a destructive and sabotaging mindset and reframing and reversing the blocks that prevent so many from moving forward. Readers will be inspired to embrace the possibility for lasting transformation. As a practitioner who works primarily with clients seeking to transform their relationship with food and their bodies, I can state that I am absolutely aligned with all

Jen speaks to in this fantastic book and will be recommending it as a valuable resource."
—Mindy Gorman-Plutzer, FNLP, CEPC, CHC, author of *The Freedom Promise*

"In reading *Diet Disruption*, I realized that I'm a mini-kitty cat who has been eating like a lion for decades. I've always thought that I should get to eat as much as anyone else because that's what's fair. Thank you for disrupting this self-sabotaging thought. I'm already implementing the straightforward strategies (for myself and my clients) laid out in this genuine and fun read."
—Heather Aardema, NBC-HWC, FMCHC, founder of Root of Wellbeing

"*Diet Disruption* will guide you back to sanity and serve up ready-to-go, realistic solutions. With characteristic compassion and deep, scientific understanding, Jen gets to the heart of the modern being with weight, eating, and worthiness. For the love of life, let *Diet Disruption* show you how to stop doing what doesn't work and start doing what does."
—Yvete Coleman, certified weight loss consultant, RTT therapist, founder of FreeForm

"It's like Jennifer knows me; my struggles were reflected on every page of this book. Unlike other weight loss books, this one gives me hope. Losing weight is a journey of personal development. This book makes what I thought was impossible very achievable."
—Di Ana Pisarri, Founder of The Parent Shift

"*Diet Disruption: The Weight Loss Solution for Chronic Serial Dieter* is a book that is long overdue. In these pages, Jennifer Powter not only demonstrates her astonishing expertise in the science of body transformation, she also engages her reader with genuine empathy and understanding so that this transformation suddenly feels wholly reachable, even for someone who has been dieting unsuccessfully for years."

—Bret Gregory,
chief customer attraction officer

"Jen makes one of the most common challenges of our time not only real and relatable, but solvable for many. Her book shines a light on the basics of nutrition and how most people become overweight. Jen truly brings it home with her ability to dive into the behavioral side of lasting weight loss in an honest and easy to relate to way. She guides readers through self-discovery and awareness, and sets them up with a method and plan to overcome the emotional side of overeating.

This book is for anyone who deeply desires to get off the psychologically and physiologically damaging journey of yo-yo dieting and lose the weight for good."

—Dr. Patricia Hort, BSc, DC,
owner and CEO of Dr. For Moms Perinatal
and Pediatric Natural Health Center

"Jennifer Powter's *Diet Disruption* gives hope to those of us who know how to lose weight but have not kept it off for the long run. She guides you to get in touch with your unique "why" that can get you to be at your ideal weight for good and feel good about yourself while loving yourself."

—Kathy Cook, M.D., dermatologist

"*Diet Disruption* is a breath of fresh air in the otherwise murky and confusing world of dieting. Jen's approach is grounded in science, tailored to the unique dietary and emotional needs of women, and based on the realities most women face day in and day out. She definitely walks the talk, and her brutally honest sharing of her own weight loss experience is both inspiration and revelation."

—J. Ross, client

"I read the entire book in one sitting. It's honest, humorous, and encouraging. The most important factors revealed are the emotional reasons why many of us struggle. As a mental health professional, I would highly recommend this book for anyone who faces challenges of not enough."

—Rosemarie Marotta, M.S., C.P.M.

"I wish I had had this book more than fifty years ago when I started my first diet at age twelve, or when I continued to deprive myself during the next five decades, constantly searching for the magic answers that would work for me through the misguided diet and exercise trends of the day. Jennifer reveals a deep understanding of the female psyche and situation and provides a compelling argument for holistic change and a sustainable way to approach weight loss and good health."

—Penny Jadwin, former chronic serial dieter

"*Diet Disruption* is a must-read for any woman on this planet that struggles with the 'why can't I' mindset around weight loss. Jennifer has a unique way of connecting with readers through her honesty, experience and science-based knowledge around dieting myths. She delivers a powerful message that any chronic dieter needs to read."

—P. Twamley, client

"Finally, someone who is telling women the truth about the dieting industry and how it has failed them! As a how-to guide, *Diet Disruption* is brimming with honest, straightforward knowledge and strategies every woman can use to overcome their past failures regarding weight loss. Jen is the real deal – no BS – and provides deep resources in this book with the whole truth about why this disruption is needed for all of us who choose to take control of our lives and lose the weight for the last time."

—A.J. Jones, client

"The diet industry is ripe for disruption, and that is precisely what Jennifer Powter does. *Diet Disruption* addresses the needs of people who, for years, have simply tolerated life carrying too many pounds or who are just plain tired of yo-yo dieting. It looks at why you have the extra weight not just how to get rid of it and provides a plan that is simple to implement and is sustainable for the long term. You will find yourself thinking, 'I wish someone had talked to me like this years ago, my life would have been so different.'"

—Melissa Warner, life-long yo-yo dieter

"I've long suspected that it was more in my head than my stomach as to why I couldn't lose weight. *Diet Disruption* confirms my suspicions and has given me some great suggestions on how to overcome these obstacles."

—Julie Wiseman, widowed mom of four kids

Ley, it has always been, and will forever be you.

I love our love.

I love you.

To all of our children, Olivia, Jacob, Sadie, Lee, Mason, and Spencer, you have brought more gifts into my life than you could ever imagine.

I am so lucky.

I love you.

Contents

1

Why Is Weight Loss So Hard?

*"A strong woman looks a challenge in
the eye and gives it a wink."*
—Gina Carey

You're a busy woman. As you were tackling life, slaying dragons, and becoming successful, you lost yourself along the way. When you look in the mirror, you don't even recognize yourself.

Your life looks good from the outside – nice husband, great children, fabulous house, cabin, cars, and you go on vacations. But you're a mess on the inside. Miserable. It feels like you're in such a life-rut and you don't understand why. You have everything you've ever wanted – except for how you look and feel about yourself.

You're overweight. Fat, if you will. You used to run and be active but you're now out of breath after a flight of stairs. "How'd I let myself get this way?" you wonder. It started after having kids. You were just so busy and tired. You never lost the baby weight and then with all of life's stresses and demands you put on even more weight. There are twenty-plus extra pounds on your body and you hate it.

It's not like you're lazy. You've done all the diets. You name it, you've tried it – Weight Watchers, Jenny Craig, Atkins, South Beach, Whole 30, plus a gazillion more. Maybe you even went keto or tried paleo for a while. Of course, all of the diets worked. You lost weight when you were on a diet but it was just so hard to stick to it. Diets are restrictive. It became more exhausting for you to be on the diet than to just be miserable with your weight. You couldn't have a social life, traveling messed things up, and it seemed that by Thursday, you lost your willpower and discipline anyway. You seem to always cheat and fall off the wagon. Then the pounds came piling back on.

You are miserable and unhappy with your body. You hate going out; you feel embarrassed. You have nothing to wear and everything you do try on looks horrible. You can't even shop in your favorite stores anymore – nothing fits you. There are five different sizes of clothes in your closet right now ranging from your "skinny" ones to your "fat" ones.

You hate being in photographs. This breaks your heart because you have few pictures of yourself with your kids. Then there's your husband. He's a good man. You were thin and fit when you met. You don't know how he can stand the sight of you or feel attracted to you in a physical/sexual way, but he seems to. He tells you he loves you and wants you. But you constantly turn him down for sex. You pretend you're asleep or tell him you're too tired. You just don't feel sexy. You don't even get undressed around him. Eventually, you know you need to have sex to fulfill his sexual needs, but you hate the experience. The lights are off. You're so self-conscious. There's no way you can be on top. That used to be your favorite but it horrifies you to think of what he sees, all your rolls, your flabby body. You just feel so gross. Your sex life is awful, and you know you're the one to blame. You've noticed he's stopped trying to initiate things. You're worried

2

he's going to go seek it elsewhere. He's not as affectionate as he used to be. No hugs or handholding, no gentle touches as he passes by. It's almost like the worse you feel about yourself the less he touches you. To be honest, you don't even talk anymore. It's like you're roommates raising kids and running a household.

You don't know what's wrong with yourself. Your friend said it was hormones – that weight loss becomes impossible at this age. You don't know about that. There are plenty of thin women walking around, so that can't be it.

You keep wondering why this is so hard for you. Your mom had weight issues. You remember her taking you to her Weight Watchers meetings when you were a teenager and you learned how to count points. You weren't even overweight back then. At least, you didn't think so. And, you were at a good weight in your twenties too, before kids. A weight that you felt sexy at, strong, confident, and fit at.

Admit it. You like food. And wine. At the end of a long day, food gives you everything you need. You get to have a break and just sit and eat and you don't have to think about anything. You don't eat all the time or binge every day. Not at all. You think you and your family eat pretty healthy. You like cooking but you don't have a ton of time for it, so often you get takeout when life gets busy and the kids have activities.

On work trips, you know you eat and drink more than you should – it's like a little escape for you from the busyness, the responsibilities. It's an easy way to forget about all of life's stresses.

You need to get back in control. It's like you've said before, "Screw it, I don't care." But deep down, you do. You know this is affecting other areas of your life. It's like your self-loathing is oozing into everything – your health, your marriage, even the relationships you have with your kids. They ask you to do things with them like go for a bike ride or pass a ball around and you always say "no." You make excuses up – too tired, your knee hurts, maybe on the weekend – but they've heard this for years. You feel guilty. Like you're a bad role model.

You feel like you're in survival mode, just doing what you need to do to get by and that you simply don't have the energy for anything more. Start another diet? You don't have the strength. Besides, the weight just comes right back on anyway. Workout? Forget it. There's no way you're putting on exercise clothes or going to a gym. That whole experience would be humiliating. You walk the dog though and that's got to count for something, right?

Let's talk about the wine and the ice cream, candy, and chocolate. You can fully admit that those items are a major way for you to numb. You look forward to that glass of wine in the evening, but it's never just one. It's always two (or sometimes three) glasses. And no matter how many times you tell yourself that you're not going to eat anything bad, you always do. You get out one square of chocolate, but then before the night is over, you've eaten the whole bar. And there are times you don't stop there; you still feel like something to eat, so you'll grab some cheese and crackers or chips. And then you feel awful. Bloated and lethargic. Irritated and disgusted by yourself. Guilt, regret, and shame seep into your soul. And after those extra bad nights, the worst part is waking up the next morning and having to get dressed.

You have *nothing* to wear. You hit snooze twice before you get up because you're exhausted. You lie there and your hands travel over your body feeling your fat, squeezing it, grabbing it, hating it. You're in a bad mood before you're even out of bed – especially the days you have to be seen. You're sure everyone is talking about how you've let yourself go. You used to *love* wearing jeans and a t-shirt, but now jeans look horrible on you and a t-shirt just clings to your rolls. Dresses? Forget it. You hate your flabby arms. You just want to hide.

"How do I get a handle on this? Why is it so difficult?" These thoughts are on repeat in your brain. You wonder what's wrong with you.

You feel like you always come last and that there's no one there to support or help you. There just never seems to be enough time or energy for you to get everything done. You're exhausted.

You feel like you're just getting by. Numb. Not sure how to feel. You don't even know if you're happy. The food takes it all away for a while. It's the best distraction.

You have all of these excuses. That it's your age. Now it's too late to get thinner and fit. Too late to change your habits. Too late to fix your marriage from falling apart.

You don't know how to do this. You don't know how to create a sustainable life for yourself as opposed to being on a diet. Dieting takes so much energy. You get results, but it's because you go to extremes: black and white. All or none. You judge yourself as being either good or bad. There's no moderation for you.

Every week, you're like, "Okay, I can do this. Just eat less," and so you count every calorie you consume on whatever new app or diet you try. You eat your boring salad for lunch, but by 3 p.m., you're starving and off to Starbucks you go for a latte and a treat – the whole time telling yourself that it can't be that bad for you and it won't matter this one time.

Lies. All lies. You're a big, fat liar to yourself and you *hate* feeling like such a failure. No matter how many good things are going on for you, your weight is like a black cloud hanging over your soul.

You feel lethargic, lazy. Your pants are getting tighter, and you're like, "Ugh, again?" Your weight is ruining your life. It impacts every area of your life because you feel like crap. You don't even want to look at yourself. And part of you just wants to say, "Forget it! I'll be happy like this," and let it go. But you can't. You just can't believe this is it. That this is how you're supposed to live. You keep trying and failing. Your weight is on your mind *all* the time. It consumes you and casts a shadow over your life.

You're at a loss. You need help. You can't do this on your own. You feel like you're stuck in such a shame/guilt cycle and you have no one to talk to about it with – no one understands.

You want to lose weight without being on some crazy diet and know you'll never regain it.

You want to stop using food and wine as your coping mechanisms after a hard day.

You want to feel sexy and attractive for both yourself and your partner.

You want to be a better role model for your kids.

You want to change.

You just don't know where to start. You feel desperate and that's the worst part because that's always when you're seduced by the new, quick weight loss thing that's out even though you know it doesn't work. How do you live your life and lose weight at the same time without feeling like you're punishing yourself?

There are tons of women just like you struggling to lose weight and feeling like all they do is fail. The biggest myth women believe is that they can and should be able to do this on their own. But why? Weight loss, nutrition, and health are some of the most complex topics out there and there is a ton of misinformation. It's not easy.

For an outer transformation to happen, you have to do your inner work. That means asking the right questions so you can truly focus on creating the right solutions. Excess weight on your body is simply a physical symptom of something that is out of alignment for you in your life. It's when you start asking the right questions like, "Why am I overweight?" or "Why do I think I need to drink wine to cope with my life?" that you start to zero in and identify what the real issues are.

The fact is, women are overweight because they overeat for either or both of the following reasons:

1. They truly don't understand the consequences of their actions and the impact that their food choices have on their body

2. They don't care about that because they're so busy using food and alcohol as a coping mechanism that emotional eating is now their habit

The dieting industry is a $70 billion industry that preys on the vulnerabilities and insecurities of women. They know that when a woman gets desperate enough, she's pretty much willing to do *anything* to lose the weight. The dieting methods/tactics that exist right now are horrible. There's everything from injections, drops, pills, powders, perfumes, and food supplements that all guarantee weight loss. And, let's face it – diets *do* work; the weight comes off. But the minute a woman stops dieting, she puts the weight right back on and more. It's a vicious cycle. It's punishing.

There's a better, simpler way. If you are truly ready to change, then change is possible, but it does mean doing it differently. It means having a willingness of spirit to trust the wisdom that is in these pages as well as your intuition. Going on a weight-loss journey can be one of the most transformative experiences of your life when done the right way. The reason for this is that wherever you go, there you are with your thoughts and feelings.

At the end of the day, it's you versus you, 24/7. Every woman needs support, information, and guidance.

When you don't feel good about yourself, it's easy to withdraw and lead a less-than-inspiring life. You feel unfulfilled, and it becomes too easy to fill that gap in your life with food. I want you to wake up to your potential and to embrace your unique gifts and strengths. I want you to be bold, brave, and courageous. I don't want you to settle or to simply feel like you're surviving. That is no way to live. You get one gift of life in this body that you're in and it's up to you to make the most out of it.

So often in this day and age, it's like a badge of honor to be running around "busy" and believing that it's okay to be last on your priority list. *It's not okay.* Women who are mothers, wives, aunts, sisters, or best friends can change the conversation around weight loss so our daughters, nieces, granddaughters, et cetera don't fall victim to the same poor self-care patterns that we and the generations of women before us did.

I want you to trust yourself and know what it takes to create a healthy relationship with yourself. It's the most important relationship that you're in, and I guarantee you're neglecting it. Losing weight isn't just about the pounds lost; it's about the woman you become along the way and the life you create for yourself. Food and booze have become acceptable, legal numbing agents to life. When you numb the difficulties, you numb the good as well.

Being overweight is painful. It takes a lot of effort to remain stuck – I'd say it takes less effort to change but the problem is that women believe that dieting is the answer and if they're not on a diet, then they don't know what else to do.

It's time to create a new lifestyle. It's time to understand what you need to be fully nourished: physically, mentally, emotionally, spiritually, and sexually. If one of those pieces is off or out of whack, there will be an emotional void. It's tempting to use food to fill it but it never works. It's a bandage on an emotional bullet wound. If you're reading this, then you know it's time to do this a different way and you're ready to go deep and truly understand that the only thing you're up against is your thoughts, knowledge, and faith. And I'm here to help. I want to give you a simple starting place that begins with being kind to yourself. Radical concept, I know. But you've already tried to hate yourself thin and it didn't work.

Women all over the world have the chance to heal what's been hurting them and start shining again. You have that chance. Now, today. The best gift you can give yourself is to experience is the brilliance of your own light. It's like a star being able to see itself and say, "Wow, I never knew how truly brilliant and beautiful I am." Our world will change when every single woman can acknowledge her brilliance, beauty, and power of her voice.

My own weight loss was a pivotal point of transformation in my life. I will never forget the constant feelings of embarrassment and shame that I existed with day-to-day. Worried about who I might run into at the coffee shop or grocery store, always being behind the camera taking pictures but God forbid I was in a picture. Pushing my husband's advances away and rejecting him. Really, I was rejecting myself. I hated my weight, hated parts of myself and pieces of my life.

All of the women that come to me have a version of this that they're experiencing in their lives. For some, they navigate divorce while raising children. For others, they cope by being a caregiver to elderly parents and burning the candle at both ends so they don't slow down on their career track. Others are stay-at-home moms who've forgotten that they have value as a woman, not just as a mom or wife. And others have let dark shadows from their past color their present – emotional, physical, and sexual abuse are real things that have happened to some of the women I work with, and it's resulted in craving safety.

If this is you, you are not alone. It's okay if you've been lost for a while or took a detour and didn't know how to get back on track. You will figure that out as you read.

And, to be honest, it feels amazing to slip on a pair of skinny jeans and a tank top and know you look good. But better than that, you *feel* good. I know this because I've lived it – let me share my story with you. It's time to learn the truth about weight loss and what it truly requires to release the weight for good.

2

Don't Worry, I Get It

"There's no force equal to a woman determined to rise."
—W.E.B. Dubois

It was a bitterly cold December day and I was out for a training run. That is a gross exaggeration. It was more like a shuffle. Even then, my heart rate was through the roof. I was the last one in my group by miles. It was so cold. The wind whipped around my face freezing the tears that were streaming out of my eyes to my cheeks. I was still suffering from pelvic floor dysfunction after having two babies, so my tights were wet and felt like they were stuck to my legs with staples. I was twenty minutes away from the warm refuge of the triathlon store where we gathered after our runs.

I felt so alone. Scared. Abandoned by life. And here I was, in -20°C weather (that's -4°F), hauling my fat, out-of-shape body for a run as it was truly the only way I thought I could lose weight and feel like "me" again.

My training coach sprinted back to me like a young gazelle. He was handsome, fit, and nice, and said, "I just wanted to see how you were doing, Jen. You're doing great. You're almost there."

I wanted to punch him in the face. Instead, I wiped away the tears before he got too close, put on a fake smile and said something dumb like, "Yeah, I'm just putting one foot after the other. You go back and get warm. I'll be there soon."

He did. He left me. I know I told him to go but I was shocked that he did. Who leaves someone who is struggling? It was so cold out and I was so tired. It's only fair to let you know that I'd never been a back-of-the-pack runner. I always used to be at the front. I'd run more than ten marathons in my twenties, pre-kids, and this whole experience was embarrassing and humbling. Who was I?

After he ran off, it was like any will that I relied on drained from me and I dropped to my knees on the icy pathway and cried. I cried and cried and cried. It was freezing out so there wasn't anybody else on the pathway – no one to check and see if I was okay. It was just me.

I call it my God moment.

As the tears of frustration and loneliness poured from my soul out of my eyes and onto my face, I looked up at the sun in the blue sky and said out loud, "Oh, my God, there has to be a better way than this."

In my head, I heard this message, "There is. But you have to choose change. The path you're on isn't serving you."

I hung my head and vowed that no matter what I did, I'd choose change. I'd never be that sad, forlorn, overweight, depressed woman on the side of a path again.

Let's go back to the beginning.

Like many twenty-somethings, I spent the majority of those years in university. I first did my undergraduate degree in exercise science and I went on to complete my master of science degree specializing in exercise physiology. I got certified as a trainer and a fitness instructor along the way. I knew a *lot* about the body, how it worked, how to train it, and how to take care of it.

To afford my schooling, I worked as a wild-land firefighter in the summers and as a waitress in the winters. I also loved to run. I ran half-marathons and marathons and not for one second did I ever worry about my weight or what to eat. Like many women in their twenties, I always thought I could lose five or ten pounds, but I didn't put much effort into it. I felt good in my skin, liked how I looked naked and felt good getting dressed.

As life does, it got more complicated as I neared my thirties. My friends were all getting married and while I didn't know where my career was going to go, the only thing I'd ever wanted to be since I was little was a mom. I married a guy. Not a great guy or someone who I was fantastically in love with, but a guy. I had convinced myself that he was "the one."

We had two beautiful children and I love them beyond the beyond. But the funny thing about motherhood is no one tells you how busy it's going to be or how many things you're going to need to sacrifice. It's like a club of secrecy. We had moved to a new city where we didn't have any family, and we moved into a new house in a new neighborhood two days after my daughter was born. While I adored being a mom, I'd never felt more alone in my life. I was also trying to build a company while they napped. My husband would go to work and I'd be a mom all day. Then after dinner, I'd start my second shift (that's what I called it) and work well into the wee hours of the night.

It didn't take long for financial pressures to rise, sleep deprivation to kick in, and frustration and loneliness to be my most familiar feelings. Oh, and I weighed forty pounds more than I did before I got pregnant the first time. How in the world did this happen? I thought that we were eating healthy. I mean, sure, there were treats here and there, but nothing crazy. I didn't binge on food.

I did drink lattes throughout the day to keep me going (I *loved* the espresso machine I got as a Christmas present, so I used it constantly), and I always looked forward to a glass of red wine and a handful of chocolate chips at night. Except, it usually wasn't just one glass. It was more like two glasses. And it wasn't just one handful of chocolate chips, it was more like three. But chocolate chips are little, right? How bad could it be? Besides, I deserved it after a long day at home.

My weight was getting to me. I was patient at first and thought that once I found a routine, it would just melt off, but it didn't. Breastfeeding didn't make one bit of difference either. I hated the idea of going to the gym even though I used to train my clients in one. I felt so out of place as the overweight, frumpy woman. I remember gathering up my courage to go one winter afternoon. I wore an ugly, old, oversized t-shirt to hide my tummy and a ball cap. I walked in, walked around, avoided eye contact with anyone, and then promptly left without doing a thing. I cried in my car.

I cut out breakfast to cut down on calories. I tried to not eat lunch, too. Back then, the "move more, eat less" philosophy was still being widely promoted. But by dinner, I was starving and had these crazy carb and sugar cravings. I'd snack on crackers or chips while cooking dinner and justify that since I hadn't eaten much earlier in the day it was okay. I gained weight doing that and felt furious. How could I practically eat nothing the day before and gain weight? I became obsessed with the scale. I would weigh myself as soon as I woke up, before I peed, after I peed, before I ate, after I ate, before I went to bed – there were some days that I stood on that scale ten times a day. I'd see wild fluctuations on it; I could gain or lose three to five pounds within hours and it frustrated me to no end.

How in the world could I go to school for so many years, have an advanced degree, be a personal trainer and exercise instructor, a certified life coach, have a whole bunch of other certifications, and be fat? I was at a loss. I remember lying on the couch while my two-and-a-half-year-old son pushed my stomach in and out and said, "Squiiishhhy, squiiishhhy," and giggled. I remember thinking of all the other women out there who were overweight and didn't have the training I did. God, if this could happen to me, it could happen to anyone, I thought. No wonder we have such a screwed-up dieting industry. After eight years in school, I didn't know what to do either.

It was my birthday and I was supposed to go out and meet my girlfriends. I looked forward to seeing them. I showered and was careful to avoid looking at myself in the mirror. I pulled a "big" pair of boyfriend jeans out of my closet, tried them on, and couldn't zip them up. They were *tight*. I ripped them off, threw them on the bed, and tried on another outfit. Then another. And another. Clothes were being ripped off of hangers and thrown on to the bed in record speed. I don't know exactly when I started to cry, but I do know that I ended curled up on the floor in the fetal position, bawling. Needless to say, I didn't go out that night. I lied and said that the kids were sick.

Where was my husband with all of this? To be honest, I'm not sure if he ever knew how horrible I felt about myself. We hadn't had sex in months; I felt gross and was certain that there was no way he could be attracted to me, so I became closed and distant to him. It was easier to reject him than to be humiliated by him rejecting me. Tension in our marriage increased. There was never any fighting but there was a deafening amount of silence. We both poured our love into our kids. They were always a bright spot. But their needs eclipsed mine. I found my self-worth in being productive around the house – washing the floor, doing the laundry. I have this crystal-clear memory of wanting to go for a walk. It was a beautiful, sunny day. And I immediately told myself that I couldn't do that, that I needed to cook dinner and get the laundry done instead. Somehow, I had completely forgotten that I mattered.

What I experienced during this time in my life is that the worse I felt about myself, the quieter I became. I lost my sense of confidence, self-esteem, and my voice. It was a slippery slope and one that I slid down and didn't even realize it. I can now only see that with hindsight.

I finally decided that what I needed to do to lose weight was physically push myself more, so I signed up for a triathlon and got a triathlon coach. This wasn't any triathlon – it was Ironman Canada, the longest distance of triathlon there is. I'd done one before having kids and I'd convinced myself that this would be the only way for me to lose weight. Go harder. Go longer. Push. The training was beyond what my untrained, postpartum body was ready for, but I was desperate to fit back into my skinny jeans. I was willing to do anything.

Then my God moment happened. That moment changed everything.

I walked my way back to the triathlon store and told my coach I was quitting the training program. He looked at me gently as I held back the tears. I told him I needed to take care of some other things first. He didn't dissuade me.

I drove home, took a shower, made a cup of tea, and snuggled my babies. I spent the next three hours pouring my heart into my journal. I uncovered and flipped over every aspect of my life. I rated my happiness, my sense of fulfillment in my marriage, my health, and by my admittance, I was failing at everything. I chose change that day. I didn't know it at the time, but when you have a come-to-Jesus moment and life brings you to your knees, it changes you. It changed me.

By finally admitting I wasn't doing so well, it cracked me open and that's what facilitated one of the most life-changing years I've ever experienced. I stopped the craziness. I shut down the company I tried to build that drained my soul. I walked instead of doing chores. I stopped drinking red wine and eating chocolate chips at night. Even though I was a trainer, I hired a trainer. Even though I was a life coach, I hired a life coach. I needed help and I was willing to go find it and receive it. I admitted to myself that I was miserable in my marriage, but I wasn't able to admit that to anyone else yet. That would be later.

I threw myself into weight loss research. I went back to my textbooks. I read every nutrition study I could find; I poured through every journal article in the *Journal of Obesity* and other peer-reviewed reference journals; I filled dozens of notebooks with my findings. I went to work in one of the best weight loss clinics my city had. I got to be mentored by one of the brightest fat loss experts in the country. I worked in a metabolic lab and studied the science of basal metabolic rate and I did a gazillion metabolic assessments on men and women of all sizes and ages. I did hundreds of body composition assessments, created hundreds of customized meal plans for clients, and I coached them to success. I was on a quest to learn more; I took every course I could that would allow me to help other people to never have to go through what I did. Along the way, I became a student of neuroscience and behavior change, habit development, cognitive behavioral therapy, and other forms of psychotherapy.

I learned. I studied. I taught. I coached.

Along the way, I had a physical transformation. In the short span of ten months, I lost forty pounds and became healthy, fit, and strong enough both physically and mentally to participate in the Ironman triathlon I had originally committed to. This experience helped me understand and live my motto of "strong body, strong mind; strong mind, strong body."

You see, excess weight on your body is just a physical symptom of emotional weight that hasn't been dealt with. For me, part of the emotional weight I had to deal with was recognizing how unhappy I was in my marriage. I finally had enough emotional strength to leave my marriage and to start a new company. It was a wild, soul-churning ride.

It's now almost ten years later, and I'm living a life that is beyond my wildest dreams and it keeps getting better. My transformative experience ignited a passion for me to help other women who are stuck, confused, lost, and being held back in their life by their weight. I am now a world-renowned weight loss expert, best-selling author, keynote speaker and influencer in the health, wellness and weight loss industry. It is a privilege to be a thought leader and change agent who is disrupting the dieting industry and teaching women of all ages and stages of life, how to get to their right weight and stay there with my science-based weight loss programs.

These programs are revolutionary as they help women become masterful in trusting themselves again and experiencing freedom with food and their body. They get to live a life where they can eat and drink whatever they want, just like I do, because they understand their choices and know how to lose weight and maintain their weight loss. There's no guilt or shame or regret. There's just knowing. I want to help you live that way too. By the way, I haven't regained a pound since losing all that weight so long ago. If I can do that, so can you.

In the next chapter I will explain how to get the most out of this book and the best way to work through the chapters. I think it's important to know where you're going and that's what this next chapter is all about.

3

Lose Weight for the Last Time

"She wasn't looking for a knight,
she was looking for a sword."
—Atticus

I think you've made a brilliant decision to pick up this book. It tells me all sorts of things about you from the get-go. You're smart. You're tenacious. You haven't given up. You're at a point in your life where you're ready and willing to do the deeper work to create a permanent transformation for yourself. You're courageous, and although you may be tentative, you're taking a bold step by veering away from the dieting industry (even though it could be said that this book is a part of that industry, I beg to differ) and the oh-so-sexy fad diets that are out there. You've wised up. You know those are only short-term solutions and you're in this for the long play. You're open to learning. You know that what you're doing isn't working for you and you're tired of feeling like you're banging your head against a brick wall. You're seeking a different way, and that's what I want to give you in this book.

I highly recommend reading this book from beginning to end. Each chapter builds on the content and lessons in the previous chapters. One of my primary goals is for you to recognize that it's not your fault the weight loss industry has failed you and that you've experienced failures along the way. All that means is you've discovered the methods that don't work for you. My end goal is that you know exactly what you need to do for permanent weight loss to happen so you can go on a weight-loss journey for the final time and fully trust that the weight is gone for good.

That's exactly what chapter 4 is all about. I present the real reasons that women lose weight but don't keep it off. These are unprecedented times that we're living in and never before has health, nutrition, fitness, or weight loss been more confusing of a topic. This chapter covers the range of environmental, phys-iological, and psychological reasons that weight loss can be so difficult.

After all of my years in this industry, I know we are asking the wrong questions and coming up with the wrong solutions. It's time to reframe this. Chapter 5 is all about freeing you from the diet industry and helping you learn what you need to do instead. For so many women, they don't know how to lose weight if they're not on a diet. It's time to say goodbye to the yo-yo dieting cycle and the all-or-none dieting mentality. I'll teach you exactly what to focus on for permanent weight loss and it doesn't involve living in a state of denial and deprivation.

That said, if losing weight was easy, we'd all be size two, and plus-size clothing stores wouldn't exist, so it's critical to under-stand why self-sabotage is part of the process. Chapter 6 will help you understand why you sabotage your progress. You'll learn why that mean voice inside your head gets loud and nasty and all of the secret reasons you're afraid to lose weight. It sounds crazy, but it's true. Fear can be a huge roadblock to success – sometimes you're just simply afraid of failing again and having to deal with the crushing disappointment you experience every time you don't reach your goal.

If dieting isn't the answer to your weight loss problem, then what is? The answer lies in looking at your habits. After all, if you're the sum of your habits and you can learn how to change those, then you have the freedom to change whatever you want in your life, including your weight. Chapter 7 is all about understanding what drives your conscious and subconscious behaviors. Sometimes you're aware of why you do what you do and other times you have no clue. I teach you a powerful framework that I learned from Charles Duhigg that has been pivotal in helping hundreds and hundreds of women lose weight and keep it off.

There are also some practical and tactical things you need to know to make your weight-loss journey easier. I want you to let go of thinking you need more willpower or discipline to be successful and instead, learn other strategies that will create smooth sailing for you to drop those unwanted pounds. The strategies in chapter 8 are often the most neglected aspects of what it takes to create a healthy lifestyle, that feels easy to live, and they are such simple tweaks. Diet books don't teach you about them, that's one of the reasons diets feel like they're so hard. They're narrowly focused. I want to expand your skillset so that weight loss gets to be easy for you.

I also want to clear up the biggest myth of weight loss: You do not need to exercise like a crazy woman. Chapter 9 will help you get clear on the role exercise needs to play in your life. Reading this chapter will lighten the load of weight loss stress you've been living under, especially if you've felt like the reason you can't ever get to your right weight is because you can't exercise due to injury, or you're just so unfit, it seems impossible that you could ever be fit and enjoy moving your body. Exercise and weight loss are like a vicious merry-go-round for some women. It goes like this, "I can't lose weight because I can't exercise. Because I can't exercise, I can't lose weight." Let's give a hallelujah for clearing up this big misconception.

The weight loss industry is a $70 billion industry that is full of companies selling pills, cleanses, supplements, teas, and other short-term, bogus solutions. Chapter 10 is all about coming back to the "weight loss basics," something that is incredibly ignored in the dieting industry. If you want to lose weight for the final time, then you cannot skip this chapter. I address the other key lifestyle components that need your attention if you want to lose weight and live with energy to thrive. If you choose to stay on the hamster wheel of life and engage in continued self-neglect, cope with high levels of chronic stress, burn the candle at both ends and live life sleep-deprived, then weight loss will never happen. That's a fact. We will explore how neglecting these areas of your life have a profound impact on your overall health and weight loss goals.

If all weight loss required was to eat less and move more, then it's probably fair to say that we wouldn't have the obesity crisis that we have in North America. But humans have feelings. Most weight gain or inability to lose weight stems from the habit of eating your feelings instead of feeling them and expressing them. Chapter 11 illustrates the addictive nature of emotional eating and will guide you to explore what you've been truly hungry for and how to give that to yourself (no food required).

As much as I need to teach the emotional eating component of weight loss, I've found there's a need to teach women about food. This is something that gets skipped over. We're barely taught this information when we're young, and if you're like most women who've been chronic dieting for years (or decades), you're suffering from mass confusion, and sometimes fear, around food.

Are carbs good or bad? Does fat make you fat or do you need fat? Is it okay to have a cheat meal or cheat day? Chapter 12 addresses the basics of food and teaches you how to understand food so you can make conscious choices with it, not cheat with it.

Going on a weight-loss journey is the most profound transformational journey a woman can take. Why? Because wherever you go, there you are. Weight loss is a you-versus-you experience. You and you alone are with the thoughts in your head, the feelings in your heart and your life experiences in your soul. I fundamentally believe that by truly choosing to change your weight, you are changing your life. In the end, it will never, ever be about the pounds lost. It will be about the life you gain, and the woman you become on this journey. Chapter 13 explains the true gifts of going on this journey and the crucial life lessons you will be blessed in experiencing in detail.

When you go on a diet, it often requires you to give up all sorts of things in your life that you like – I don't just mean food. I often hear women saying that they can't go out with their friends or go on dates because "it ruins their diet" or "they blow it." Chapter 14 explores all of the real-life challenges that women face when they stop dieting and instead choose to lose weight for the final time in a healthy, permanent way. This focuses on the mindset you need to adapt to be successful and the possible weight loss hijackers that will come along and how you can handle them.

Lastly, chapter 15 will ignite your inner hope and excitement that you can lose weight for the final time and keep it off. Faith in yourself and your ability to do this will be restored and your confidence will be renewed. Yes, you can do this. You will finally have a thorough understanding of why you've failed in the past, how you can correct that and move forward with gusto – like Sonya did.

Sonya came to one of my two-day live Weight Loss Workshops with her friend June. June happened to see an ad for this event on Facebook and immediately called up Sonya asking her to go with her. She said, "sure," without truly knowing what she was saying yes to – don't you just love those kinds of friends?

I remember seeing Sonya from the stage. She was in the second row and sat with her arms crossed and a flat expression on her face. She was short, in her mid-forties, had brown hair and was dressed in black. When she looked at me, her expression was guarded but when she talked with her friend and mingled with the other women at the event she was quick to laugh, had a beautiful smile and her eyes would light up. But she would shut down just as quickly.

Several times during the day I noticed her using the tissues on the table – dabbing at her eyes, wiping her nose. My live events are emotional – I help women get in touch with the feelings that they've been ignoring for years and come to terms with their weight, their health, their life so I'm never surprised if there are tears. It was near the end of day one that Sonya volunteered for the "hot-seat" coaching on stage. It takes courage to do this as you're now in front of the whole room sharing the most vulnerable parts of yourself.

Sonya told me that she was 5'1", weighed 215 pounds, had just been diagnosed with diabetes and was worried about the state of her health. She was a single mother who raised her daughter on her own, was a self-proclaimed workaholic, and hadn't dated in almost twenty years. She got divorced when her daughter was a baby and had put all of her energy into her child and career. Sonya was a key sales manager in a huge company and ran her division like a boss – she was bright, compassionate and highly respected. She told me that she *hated* her weight and had tried numerous things to get "rid of it" including Bernstein.

The Bernstein diet is a medically supervised program where you get injections and are required to live on an exceptionally low calorie, low carb, no fat diet (700 to 900 calories per day).

She'd done Bernstein three times and each time she'd lose twenty to thirty pounds, but then she'd regain everything she'd lost plus more. She was at her heaviest yet and her latest doctor's appointment scared her. She was literally at a loss about what to do. What she had tried in the past had made her feel like a failure, her weight had ballooned, she was confused with all of the conflicting diet information out there and so she'd remained frozen and in denial and had somehow found herself at my live event.

By following the principles that I'm about to share with you in this book Sonya, who you'll hear about again in chapter 14, created the transformation of a lifetime. To date she's lost almost thirty pounds, her doctor took her off her diabetes medication, she's started dating, she created boundaries in her work and now has a much more reasonable schedule. Most importantly, she lives life feeling joyful every day and good in her skin.

The reality of being able to feel free with both food and your body is so close, and now you get to believe that you too can experience life living this way. If I can do it, so can you. If hundreds and hundreds of my clients can do it, so can you. You've got this.

4

It's Not Your Fault

"I can and I will. Watch me."
—Carrie Green

If you're like most overweight women I know, you carry a ton of shame and guilt about your weight and even more about your inability to lose weight and keep it off. Every time you try a new diet and see the number on the scale decrease, you feel great. But then you stop the diet and the weight comes piling back on, sometimes even more than you originally lost. It feels humiliating. It makes you want to hide. It's scary. It can feel like no matter what you do, this struggle is always going to be something that you carry around and fail at.

The painful part of all of this is that with each new diet you try and with each failure, the mean, negative self-talk gets worse. The level of shame increases as does the hopelessness.

I get it. I want you to know that it's not your fault.

We are living in unprecedented times and the whole world of health, nutrition, weight loss, fitness, and diets has never been more confusing. Along with that, there's never been such incredible access to food in first world countries. Some drive-throughs are open twenty-four hours a day. Most people live within two miles of a convenience store. You can get food delivered all hours of the day and night. It's there when you want it and even when you don't. Food is available twenty-four hours a day, seven days a week.

Fifty years ago, this wasn't the case. Access to food was limited and so were resources. If you think about your grandparents or your great grandparents, they didn't have dessert every single night. It just wasn't available. It takes time to make a cake or cookies. It required ingredients like butter and sugar that were expensive and less available back then. Now, you can go to a grocery store at 10 p.m. and put cookies, cake, and a pie into your cart.

Your metabolism has not kept up with the rate of availability of food.

To be clear, your metabolism refers to a series of chemical processes by which the food you eat turns into fuel to keep you alive. Basal Metabolic Rate (BMR) is the measurement of how many calories your body needs while doing nothing. All of the cells in your body require energy to function and properly do their jobs. People talk about metabolism like it's something they can easily influence and control but that's just not the case.

Perhaps you've read blogs or articles that talk about how eating spicy foods, drinking coffee, or consuming different "metabolic boosting" supplements "speed up your metabolism." The truth is, that change is so negligible and short-lived (less than a day) that there is no way it can ever positively impact your weight loss. If it were true, we'd all be munching and crunching on jalapeño or red hot chili peppers all day long, in spite of the burn.

Your metabolism is directly influenced by your gender, age, body composition and activity level and the easiest way to explain this is the bigger you are and the more muscle you have, the higher your metabolism will be. The higher or bigger or faster (these words are often used interchangeably to describe a "good" metabolism) your metabolism is, the more calories your body needs to stay alive, which means you can eat more. The truth is, there is no such thing as "good" metabolism – there's just a metabolism that is *normal* for the above components (gender, age, body composition). And, even those with higher metabolisms are at risk of gaining weight if they consume more calories than their body needs.

Because we live in a world where there is such unlimited access to food, in order to eat the way we do, and not have it impact our waistlines, we'd need to be at least seven feet tall, and muscular. That is what I mean when I say your metabolism hasn't kept up with the availability of food. Instead, you need to work with the body you've got, and learn how to nourish it accordingly.

Then, there's the whole food production issue. Processed foods were not originally designed to be consumed every day; they were created for convenience at a time when many women were going into the workforce (back in the fifties after the war). But these foods tasted good and they were quick – two bonuses. A whole new industry around food was created but it was not done with your health or waistline in mind.

Michael Moss wrote an amazing book called, "Salt, Sugar, Fat" and in it he shares details of a famous meeting that occurred in April 1999, organized by the officials at Pillsbury and Kraft, that changed everything. Eleven CEOs of the major food companies (think Nestle, Nabisco, Coca Cola, General Mills, et cetera) gathered in Minneapolis for a secret meeting. This was unheard of as many of these companies were direct competitors. As a group, they employed 700,000 employees and were responsible for $280 billion in annual sales. But the health data of the United States was out and things were not looking good. Obesity and diabetes had risen at an alarming rate during the past two decades and a man named Michael Mudd, senior vice president of Kraft believed that the ingredients that they put into their convenience foods were part of the problem. To be specific, the *amount* of sugar, fat, and salt that were added to process foods was hurting the country.

Michael Mudd did a 114 slide PowerPoint presentation out-lining the risks to the public and stated that perhaps it was time for moral responsibility to play a role in how their food prod-ucts were produced so the health impact on the public wasn't so horrible. He got through most of his presentation and then took a stand asking for the other CEOs to agree with him and to come together to unite on this issue.

Silence.

Then one man spoke. Stephen Sanger, CEO of General Mills (producer of cereals like Lucky Charms, Count Chocula and many other sugar-filled breakfast products) said it wasn't their responsibility at all to care about public health. "Don't talk to me about nutrition." He said his responsibility was to produce food products that the public wanted to consume and if these products contained tons of sugar, fat, or salt, then it was on the consumer to not purchase the product.

This meeting occurred about twenty years after the war on fat began. Cardiovascular disease was on the rise in the sixties and seventies and the U.S. Government felt it needed to do something about it so in 1977, *The Dietary Goals for The United States* was published and contained dietary recommendations that were supposed to improve the health of Americans. They did anything but that. In fact, this gave permission to food companies to promote their sugar-filled products as fat-free.

Many studies had come out by this point and the research indicated that sugar was playing a direct role in obesity and diabetes but these food giants had power and it would take almost three more decades before sugar became a national focus for consumer awareness.

Perhaps if you grew up in the eighties like me, you recall that all of a sudden everything was labeled as fat-free. There was low-fat and no-fat yogurt that had as much sugar in it as a chocolate bar but somehow we were eating that for breakfast. I distinctly remember being a teenager and buying a bag of red licorice and thinking I was eating something healthy as it was labeled "fat-free."

People consumed sugar at a free-for-all rate thinking that it wasn't bad, but they weren't eating eggs because of the "fatty yolk." This is when a huge amount of fear and confusion around food sank in.

The dieting culture was born.

Low fat. Low cal. Very low fat. Extremely low cal. Low-carb. No carb. Atkins. Paleo. Keto. South Beach. HCG. Bernstein. Pills. Powders. Supplements. Enemas. Intermittent fasting. Vegetarian. Vegan. Omit some foods. Omit a total food group.

Restrict. Deprive. Deny. Take away. Don't have. *Can't* have.

The $70 billion dieting industry.

Worldwide, more than 1.9 billion adults (eighteen years or over) and more than 381 million children (less than eighteen years old) are overweight according to the World Health Organization. Of that, approximately 40 percent of women are classified as obese. Women are desperate to lose weight and will do almost anything to get the weight off. Perhaps you have even jumped from diet to diet to diet over the past few years. One stat I read said that women will spend twenty-five years of their life dieting. That's a long time to spend suffering, and feeling the shame, guilt, and humiliation of never being successful or reaching your goal. With all of the different diets out there it's not surprising that there are a plethora of diet myths too.

Here are the top five weight loss myths my clients have fallen victim to.

Myth #1: Eat Less So You Can Lose More

This goes hand-in-hand with skipping meals and grabbing a coffee to try to get through the day. The problem with this is when you go all day with nothing in you, you're way more likely to overeat the next time you do have a meal. You're also more likely to grab high-calorie snacks or things loaded with sugar as you have these intense cravings and in that moment, hunger wins. This is a point that some even say, "Forget about it. I'm going to do whatever I need to do right now and I'm going to start my diet again tomorrow or on Monday."

The other challenge with trying to skip meals and not eat much is you feel horrible both physically and emotionally. Physically you can experience things like headaches, fatigue, lack of energy, and emotionally you're simply not able to adequately deal with the stressors in your life. It's not uncommon for a woman who is dieting to experience mood swings irritation, frustration, anger outbursts, impatience, anxiety, and despair. Often, this is simply because you're just not nourishing your body or yourself the way you need to.

The problem with this is that it becomes a habit to not eat. You don't feel hungry in the morning or at lunch because you've become so disconnected with what your body needs that you can't even tune into your actual biological hunger signals because you've learned to ignore them.

Myth #2: Carbs Are Bad and Make You Fat

This is a blanket statement that is simply false. Carbohydrates were first demonized by the popular Atkins diet back in the seventies and have once again been vilified by keto and paleo fans. Perhaps understanding exactly what carbohydrates are can prevent you from being fearful of them. Carbs are one of the three primary building blocks of your diet, along with protein and fat, which provide your body with energy. Carbs, protein, and fat are commonly referred to as "macronutrients," while vitamins and minerals are classified as "micronutrients."

Carbs come in simple forms like sugar and in complex forms like starch and fiber. Both sugars and starch break down into glucose in your body, a simple sugar that the body uses to feed its cells whereas fiber can't be digested and passes through your body.

Here are the three main groups:

1. Sugars – this is considered a simple form of energy as it's a short-chain compound (only one or two molecules) and it breaks down to glucose easily in the body and quickly. Sugars can occur naturally in fruit and some veggies but it is also easily created and is added to many foods (white sugar, brown sugar, honey, molasses – there are over fifty names for sugar nowadays).

2. Starch is a complex form of sugar as it's composed of many molecules strung together. It takes longer to break down in the body and is considered a slower release of energy (think of things like brown rice, oats, or quinoa).

3. Fiber is found in a variety of whole foods like fruit, vegetables, whole grains, and legumes.

The problem with carbs is that we *overeat them*. Eating too much of anything can make you gain weight but it's particularly easy to eat more carbs than we need. Why? Because they taste good. They break down into simple sugars in our body and can give us that sugar-high. It's easy to grab-n-go with carbs. Think about it – chocolate, crackers, granola bars, juice, pop, chips, muffins, bagels, pastries, cookies. These are all carbohydrate-based foods. They're easy to eat. But you don't just eat four crackers, you eat ten. Chocolate bars are sold often as king-sized bars these days. You may not intend to eat both but you do. Eating a muffin from a bakery is equivalent to eating 500 calories or a Big Mac from McDonalds. Carbs are dense, meaning they pack a huge caloric punch in a small volume of food. Trying to get full by just eating carbs is a recipe for failure and a guaranteed recipe for weight gain.

When you eat carbohydrates appropriately, meaning within the right serving sizes and amount for your body, they don't make you fat. Carbs are considered a healthy, essential part of your diet. It's when you overeat them or use them as your favorite emotional eating go-to food that you get into trouble.

Myth #3: Diet Foods Can Help Me Lose Weight

Let's give props to the diet industry for creating a whole new category of foods: "diet food." Typically diet foods are supplement based, chemically created, come in a bag, box, wrapper, or container and are designed to fool you into thinking weight loss will be achievable this way, while making the creators of said food products wealthy. If you've ever relied on two shakes a day and a bar to live off of, you know what I mean. It can make you feel like a crazy person around food. There are so many food products out there that are marketed as "low-fat" or "no-fat," which instantaneously make us think we won't gain fat if we eat them and often they're loaded with sugar or salt. Things can be gluten-free, farm-fresh, organic and yet you can still overeat them.

Diet foods are part of the worldwide weight loss problem that exists. It's time to switch the focus from "dieting" to nourishing yourself and learning how to do that by eating real food, in the right quantities for the right reasons. When this is accomplished you won't need "diet food" anymore because you've finally created a healthy relationship with real food.

Myth #4: Overweight People Have Slow or Broken Metabolisms

I can't tell you the number of times I've talked to a distressed, overweight woman on the phone who is sure that the reason she can't lose weight is because her metabolism is *slow* or *broken*. Perhaps if I hadn't worked in a metabolic lab measuring metabolisms I'd be sucked in by this claim, but I know better and the research shows us this just isn't true. In fact, most people who weigh more are more likely to have a higher or faster basal metabolic rate, not a slower one because they have more skeletal muscle on their frame. Your body had to adapt and create more muscle so you could continue to move around. The real reasons you're overweight are much more likely to be due to emotional eating, distracted eating, and overeating for your size.

That said, in some cases, there are legit medical causes for a slower metabolism which shouldn't be ignored. Factors such as hormonal imbalances, thyroid dysfunction, and some prescription medications can influence metabolic function. I always recommend consulting your physician at the beginning of your weight-loss journey.

Myth #5: You Need to Do a Cleanse or Detox to "Kickstart" Weight Loss

The reason Weight Loss Cleanses and Detoxes are so popular is they give you a "start" date. You have a plan, a set time frame that you're going to commit to something and there are strict rules to follow. And somehow, in your brain, you start to believe that you can go twenty-one days with just liquids, and that it makes sense to use enemas. So, you go "all-in" until you start to feel faint and can't think straight and decide that you'll re-commit next Monday instead. And you feel disappointed because you did just lose three pounds, but the truth is that that weight loss will be short-lived.

Cleanses and detoxes are trendy because they seem like a simple, fast solution and that's the problem. True weight loss happens and is sustained when you do the work to create a lifestyle with food and your habits that you can enjoy and live with. Fact is, if you can't see yourself doing this in five years then you're on a diet. And it won't work, not in the long run.

Kitty Cat versus a Lion

One of the things that I teach at my live events and to my clients is the concept of being a kitty cat versus being a lion. Stay with me here, this is important. I want you to think of a kitty cat – I'm talking about a cute, little, domestic house cat. Hold that image in your mind. Now, I want you to think of a lion. Chances are you've seen a lion at the zoo, on a nature show, or in a picture. It's a huge, beautiful, powerful, muscular animal, right? In your mind, see those two animals, which are the same species, side by side. Now let me ask you which animal needs to eat more food: the cat or the lion? This isn't a trick question.

The lion needs to eat more. Why? Because it's a bigger animal. It requires more nutrients to sustain its life.

What would happen if the kitty cat ate as much as the lion? It would become a fat cat. The cat would be eating way beyond what its little body requires. Even though the cat and the lion are from the same species, the cat simply does not need as much food as a lion does. The kitty cat has perfect physiology for its size. Its body isn't broken. It doesn't have a bad metabolism. The cat would simply be overeating for its metabolic demands and the cat's body would store all of that excess consumption of food as fat.

You, my beautiful friend, are a kitty cat and you are living in a lion-sized world. And it has created enormous confusion for you. Restaurants serve lion-sized portions. Plates, bowls, and wine glasses are designed for lions. If you're married or have a boyfriend, you're living with a lion. Men tend to be bigger than women. They are typically taller and have more muscle mass which means they get to eat like lions.

When you have the metabolism of a kitty cat and eat like a lion, you get fat. That is why you are overweight. Chances are you've been taking lion-sized portions, on lion size plates and haven't even realized it. you do what most women do, and you start to blame your body. You start to believe that your body is broken. You start to believe that you must have a bad or slow metabolism. You might even be blaming hormones or the stage of life that you're in (like perimenopause or menopause). You start to feel betrayed by the fact that your body isn't working for you. And then you diet to lose weight. The devastating cycle of dieting begins.

The human body is a brilliant machine. Think of it – your heart beats, your blood circulates, you breathe, you digest food, and, as a woman, you can even create life. Your body has innate intelligence and wisdom. When you eat with a lack of understanding of how much your body needs to sustain your life, if you engage in emotional eating, if you eat lion-sized portions, if you eat without paying attention or understanding the implications of your choices, then all of that excess energy that your body doesn't need must be converted into something. Your body takes that excess energy that you don't need and stores it as fat.

Lack of Knowledge Around Food

One of the things that I help my clients most with is being able to understand food. For so many women, one of the basic problems is that you just don't understand how your body works and the consequences of the food choices that you're making. You're simply unaware. In the past thirty years or so, carbohydrates have gotten a bad rap. From Atkins to paleo to keto, women have become afraid of eating carbohydrates, and, let's face it. we live in a big carbohydrate-based world. It can feel like almost everything is a carbohydrate. You've been taught that eating bread and pasta and rice is what makes you fat. But it's a lot more complicated than that, or is it?

It's Time to Dig up the Dandelion

I remember when I owned my first home and took pleasure in taking care of the yard. I loved the green grass. When I would see a dandelion pop up, I would just pluck the yellow head off so I could continue to see a field of green when I looked out my window. But, sure enough, the dandelion would pop back up again with a yellow head, sometimes two. And, the dandelions spread. Before long, I had a backyard full of dandelions. A lot of people suggested to just use RoundUp, but I felt horrible about the idea of poisoning the earth. I wanted to find a different way.

I asked my mom how to get rid of dandelions. She gave me a strange look and said, "Honey, you need to get to the dandelion root. You can't just pluck the head off. You need to dig down deep in the soil and dig out the root out or else the dandelions are just going to keep coming back."

Ah. Problem solved. It took some time, and it was a lot more work than just plucking off the yellow heads, but with persistence, I was able to dig up all of those dandelions and had a lawn full of green grass again.

I bring this up because dieting is like trying to pluck off the dandelion head when there's a deeper issue. Let's think about that. The dandelion head is above the ground. It's easy to see. It's bright yellow, and you want it gone. That's just like your weight. It's visible. You hate it, and you want it to go. You try superficial tactics like dieting. You try restricting calories. Omitting food groups. You try short-term solutions like cleanses and detoxes because it simply seems easier. But just like that dandelion in my backyard, the weight keeps coming back, and sometimes it's more than what it was before. The issue has gotten bigger.

You have to recognize that your weight is a symptom of something deeper going on. You may not even recognize or know what those deeper root issues are. The kind of root issues I'm talking about are things like living with loneliness, boredom, anger, resentment, anxiety, fear, or feeling lost or uninspired. Hating your job, your relationship, or your financial situation. Maybe the years or decades of living with chronic stress have simply become your new "normal" and being unhappy has become a way of existing.

At some point, you may have told yourself that you simply needed to suck it up or deal with it. That this was all that you are going to get to have in your life. Maybe you feel like things are pretty good and some people have it worse than you so you should just be happy with what you've got. Except you're not. Any of those root issues above could be the reason that you engage in overeating or mindless eating. I talk about this later in the book. But it's time to get real now.

I deeply believe that if you are currently facing a weight loss challenge, then you've been given a gift. Life is asking you to wake up and pay attention. The days of self-neglect are over. The days of not even knowing how to prioritize your needs and wants so that you can feel happy and fulfilled are done. If you are reading this, then your heart of hearts self is begging you to take a different path and to get to the root issues in your life. It's time. The biggest myth women tell themselves is that they'll take care of this when they have more time or feel less busy or when the kids are older or when work isn't so crazy, and decades of your life can slip by.

If you have been a chronic dieter or living a binge/restrict lifestyle with food, you may believe that change is hard. Well, dieting is hard. Living your life with no freedom, feeling restricted by what you can or can't have, feeling deprived of never being able to have the foods that you enjoy is hard. Living life feeling depressed and anxious, hating your body, hating yourself – that's hard.

What you have to realize is that your emotional energy is getting spent anyway. The energy of feeling stuck, the energy of feeling less-than, of never wanting to go out, the energy that you give to hiding yourself and being engaged in self-loathing – that is soul-sucking energy. It's truly depleting. The energy that you expend to create positive change is equal to the energy that you are going to spend if you choose to stay stuck in a dieter's rut. I don't know about you, but I'd way rather spend my energy on creating the life that I want and doing the work to dig up the root issues so I can create permanent change in my life.

One of the biggest problems is that women get caught in the comfort trap. Think about it: how many times have you heard that we're creatures of comfort? Maybe you like the comforts of home or comfort food and the biggest challenge that you are going to face is being willing to get uncomfortable.

If you're not uncomfortable, then you're not changing.

Change requires you to go from what feels familiar and secure, even if you don't like it, to the unfamiliar, the unknown.

Often, focusing on your weight loss challenges is the most effective distraction you have from paying attention to the rest of your life. It's easier to look for the next diet than it is to ponder whether or not you're happy in your marriage. It's easier to go keto then it is to decide to quit your job and go after your passion. It's easier to drink a bottle of wine at night instead of admitting to yourself that you're unhappy and feel lonely. I get it. That's why I know going on a weight-loss journey will be the most transformative journey of your life. It's not about the weight that you lose. Sure, it's nice to fit into an amazing outfit or a pair of skinny jeans or that sexy little black dress, but really, the true accomplishment is in the woman that you get to become.

Transformation is not for the faint of heart. It requires courage, tenacity, persistence, and support. Going on a diet is a superficial tactic like trying to pluck off the yellow dandelion head and hoping the dandelion will never come back. Committing to a weight-loss journey is about becoming willing to get to your root issues and to go into the deep dark areas of your life that scare you.

This means you can no longer hold faulty expectations of your body. This means you can no longer believe the crazy misinformation that you read on tabloid magazines like, "Lose your baby belly in ten days" or "Drop thirty pounds in two weeks." It means you have to be strong enough to resist the temptation to do something quickly because quick weight loss leads to quick weight regain. You've been there, you've done that, you know this to be true. Permanent weight loss is going to be slower than you want it to be. I get that. I know you're impatient. Chances are your self-esteem and self-confidence are at all-time lows at this moment. But if those approaches had worked for you, you wouldn't be reading this book right now.

Let's talk about healthy weight loss expectations for a moment. You've probably read the general stat which says losing roughly two pounds a week is good. Here's the zinger: if you're 5'4" or under, that would be exceptional weight loss and probably only achieved through dieting. If you're a woman who's more petite, then you've probably noticed that weight seems to come on quicker and takes longer to lose. That's because you're like a mini kitty cat. Weight loss is different for you. The journey will take longer. You will require more patience with the process. But don't worry, all of my clients who are 5'4" and under, achieve freedom with the food, which means you can too.

My whole approach is that you don't need to diet. You simply need to understand your body and the impact of your food choices, and from that create a lifestyle that you love and can enjoy for the rest of your life.

My clients don't talk about being on a program or dieting when they work with me. The nature of saying that you're "on" something means that you could be "off" something and that takes you to the "on-the-wagon-off-the-wagon-dieting" philosophy. Instead, you and I are going to talk about choices and results. The first thing I want to teach you is that you don't need to rely on willpower and discipline to reach your goals. Instead, I want to show you some simple ways that you can truly set yourself up for a lifetime of success with losing weight one last time and then keep it off forever.

I truly believe it's not your fault if your weight has crept up and you haven't had success with diets in order to lose the weight for good. They're not designed for you to be successful in the long term. But now that you know what you're up against with the 24/7 availability of food, and the food production companies not caring about your health, only their profits, then it is your responsibility to take a stand for yourself and truly decide what you want. Knowing the right info is critical, and being able to recognize the most common weight loss myths out there means you're arming yourself with knowledge so you don't fall victim to any bright, new, shiny diet that pops up. One of the pieces of information in this chapter that I urge you to commit to is eating like the kitty cat you are; often this change alone can create a surprising release of weight that felt easy to do – and of course that makes sense, you don't have to diet, just pay attention to your portions and own the choices you're making.

The reason to pay close attention to what comes next in the following chapter is so you can finally ditch your fat clothes for good. You'll no longer need to keep five different sizes of clothes in your closet or live with constant fear around food or continually feel stressed that the weight is going to come back because you will no longer be engaged in the yo-yo diet cycle. That's right – you're about to break up with the "good/bad" "on-the-wagon/off-the-wagon" dieting mentality that has kept you trapped in a body you've been at war with for years.

5

Kiss the Yo-Yo Dieting Cycle Goodbye

"She was on a journey that required her to be fierce. She was up for the task."
—Unknown

I believe that to find an answer to a problem, we need to understand what the problem is. For most women, they think that the problem is that they're overweight and so they try to figure out how not to be. They focus on losing weight.

It's time to start asking better questions to find better solutions.

The typical question is, "What am I going to do to lose weight?" I think you should be asking, "What caused me to gain weight in the first place?" If you don't know why the weight came on, how do you ever expect to lose it and keep it off?

You already know that dieting is not the answer, not in the long run. I mean, sure, any diet can cause you to lose weight while you're on it, but what happens the minute you stop dieting? You gain all of the weight back and then some. Think back to all of the different diets you have tried and how they made you feel. If you're like most of my clients, being on a diet has caused you to live life feeling deprived and in a constant state of anxiety. Not to mention hungry, frustrated, tired, emotionally exhausted, confused, anxious, and fearful of food. This chapter dives deep into the real reasons you overeat, how to distinguish between true hunger and emotional hunger, what emotional hunger is and better ways to cope with the "witching hours" when you *feel* like something to eat but aren't hungry.

The typical dieting mentality looks something like this:

- You're either on a diet or off a diet
- You're "on the wagon" or "off the wagon"
- You're either "good" or "bad"

It's such rigid thinking. It feels strict and there are usually a lot of rules to follow in terms of what you're allowed to eat and what you can't have. It's like living in a perpetual state of denial and deprivation. And, the minute you're told you can't have something do you notice that you want it even more? You may even start to obsess or fantasize about that food and think about how, when you're at your goal weight, you're going to eat as much of that food as you want. You plan it out.

Being a chronic dieter has harmful psychological consequences. You no longer trust yourself, have a fear of food, and body image issues. Living in a perpetual state of denial and deprivation can lead to overeating and bingeing – fact.

The dieting industry is a $70 billion industry that preys on the insecurities of women. The marketing budgets of these companies are huge, and they know that when you feel bad enough about yourself, when you get desperate enough – you're willing to do almost anything to lose the weight *fast*, and so, fast weight loss is what they promise. Even driving around my city, I've seen signs offering women a chance to freeze their fat off, to lose thirty pounds in thirty days (guaranteed), and other crazy things.

The Yo-Yo Diet Cycle

Nancy, who is sixty-three, is the principal of a big high school. She's highly-educated and extremely committed to her job. She came to me during a break at one of my two-day live events in tears. Nancy told me about how for the past fifty years she'd been in a vicious yo-yo diet cycle. It started when she was a young girl, just eight years old. Her mother took her to her doctor and asked that he put Nancy on a diet. She said that she didn't want a fat daughter. Looking back, Nancy was able to see the shame and humiliation she experienced in that office and knows that was the beginning of her lifelong weight struggles.

She knew that she couldn't stand to do another diet but she didn't know what else to do. Nancy said that she was scared she was going to be stuck in a body that she hated for the rest of her life and she was worried about her health. She loved to travel with her husband but her weight was causing problems. She couldn't walk and hike the way he did. Her weight limited the activities they did together and she didn't want him to leave her behind.

She listed the diets that she had done in the past decade, which included being on Weight Watchers numerous times, signing up for Jenny Craig, trying Whole 30, and even trying to do keto. The latest diet that she'd been on and off over the past two years was the HCG diet – a low-fat, low-density diet that required Nancy take HCG drops and eat 500 calories a day for about three to six weeks. "I always lose weight on that but I'm miserable. I have no energy, I can barely think and I start to fantasize about all of the foods I'm going to eat once I'm at my goal weight." She rolled her eyes and hung her head. "I know how ridiculous this all sounds. I'm smart yet so stupid. I'm exhausted by this." She said, "I'm always so good at the beginning. I'm able to do it 100 percent but after I lose fifteen or twenty pounds I'm less committed. I let work get in the way. My job is stressful – there's always treats from parents in the staff room and I eat them telling myself that I deserve them because I'm working so hard. I tell myself that this just isn't a good time, or that this isn't working and I let myself off the hook. I just seem to oscillate between these crazy extremes and I don't know what else to do."

I gave Nancy a huge hug and told her I completely understood. She was engaged in yo-yo dieting and was fighting a battle she was never going to win unless she became willing to do something differently. She said she was ready.

Yo-yo dieting is when you engage in short-term changes regarding what you eat and how you move your body. That means the results are also short-term. It looks something like this. You're out at an event and someone snaps a picture of you. You see it, and it's shocking. You wonder, "Is that me? Oh, my gosh, how did this happen?" The shame and self-loathing feelings kick into high gear. You decide, "That's it. I'm going on a diet." You don't care what you do; you're willing to do anything, it doesn't matter how ridiculous or hard or restrictive the diet sounds, you'll do it.

You do some research that night staying up late to find the thing that's going to work. Maybe you go to the health food store the next day and buy the latest twenty-one-day cleanse that you read a celebrity is doing or your best friend did and she lost ten pounds. You go home and feel a brief moment of relief because you've started something.

The first *yo* of the yo-yo diet cycle is when you decide that you're no longer going to eat anything that's not good for you. Say goodbye to chocolate, cheese, chips, ice cream, cookies, wine, even beets, carrots, and bananas because you heard they have too much sugar in them. You tell yourself that you're going to be just fine living on something stupid like 800 calories a day and that you like boiled chicken, eggs, and lettuce with no dressing. This is exactly what Nancy did when she was taking HCG. She kept her caloric intake under 500 calories a day and didn't let herself eat *any* of the foods she enjoyed. She constantly felt like she was depriving herself.

Going on a diet, cleanse, or detox typically puts you into a dramatic state of undereating. What's crazy is every blog post or magazine article puts generalized information out there that women of all sizes try to follow. If you're 5'8" or taller and trying to live on 1,200 calories, you will not last long. I promise. Same as if you're 5'2" and taking the recommendation to keep your caloric intake to 1,500 calories, you might not lose any weight at all and get so completely frustrated by that. Cookie-cutter programs don't work. Period.

You're able to white-knuckle this diet for a week, maybe two, and a long diet stretch might be up to three weeks, but eventually, life gets the better of you and you say, "Screw it." And then you swing the other way, which creates the other *yo* in the yo-yo diet cycle. This swing in the other direction is when you say things to yourself like, "I'm a good person, I deserve to be happy, I'm just going to eat and drink whatever I want right now and worry about this later" or, "Obviously, there is something wrong with me. No matter what I do, I can't seem to lose weight, so I might as well just eat and drink and not care." Nancy swung hard this way. She would eat the cookies and treats that parents brought in, stop at the drive-through on her way home to get fries, enjoy late-night chocolates while doing work, and justified everything she ate due to how much she'd previously restricted herself from eating these foods while she was on her short-lived diet.

When you're in the first swing of the yo-yo cycle, you are undereating for what your body requires and you can see a lot of weight come off. But what kind of weight are you losing

– is it fat? Maybe a little, but it's most likely going to be a big reduction in water weight due to changing your diet so quickly and cutting out carbs, booze, and processed foods.

When you say, "Screw it" and decide that you're going to eat and drink whatever you want, you go into a phase of total overeating for your body. Your body is smart. It's storing all of that excess caloric consumption as fat. The yo-yo diet cycle is dramatic shifts between undereating and overeating which creates weight loss and weight gain. And that's exactly what Nancy's body did. It would release the weight when she was undereating it and then pack it all back on again when she was overeating, creating this horrible weight loss/weight gain cycle that made her feel like a crazy woman.

Those are the physiological consequences of engaging in yo-yo dieting. But what about the psychological consequences. Most of my clients say things like:

- I'm exhausted; I don't want to spend the rest of my life battling food.
- I doubt myself. I'm afraid. It's so hard. I don't have any willpower left.
- This feels hopeless.
- I'm miserable. I'm miserable to be around. I'm grumpy, snappy, irritable – all of my energy goes into thinking about this.
- My weight consumes me; it's on my mind all the time.

All of the above were sentiments that Nancy expressed too, but the hardest part she said was feeling like such a failure. I helped Nancy learn how to break free from her addictive cycle of yo-yo dieting. To date she's lost forty-five pounds and for the first time in her life she feels confident that she's lost the weight for good. She's traveled to Mexico with her husband, gone hiking in the mountains, and the challenge is now for her hubby to keep up with her.

Most women understand that dieting has harmful physiological consequences such as increased risk for heart disease and osteoporosis, hormone dysfunction, hair loss, electrolyte imbalances, decreased coordination and loss of muscular strength and endurance, et cetera, but often the psychological damage gets ignored. It simply becomes normal to live with the above feelings. That's why the dieting culture needs to be changed. Women deserve better than this. You deserve better than this. You deserve to know what to do so that you can have freedom with food and your body.

You don't need to diet. You need to stop overeating for your kitty cat body size and learn how to give yourself the nourishment that you need. Period. End of story.

So, that leads to this question: "Why do I overeat?"

The Reasons Women Overeat

Women overeat for a million reasons, but I'm going to present with you with the two most common ones. The first is you simply don't understand how much food and the kind of nutrients your body needs and the second is that food has become an emotional coping mechanism for you.

The first one is easy. Not everybody goes to university to get a degree in nutrition science, dietetics, or health science, and it's not like we go to "health school" in our adult years. There's simply a big knowledge gap between what you're doing and the impact that it's having on your weight. My guess is that you're brilliant at what you do. Me? I'm great with food and the body and behavior change. I went to school for almost eight years to learn about it and have continued to take advanced training during most of my adult life. But ask me about taxes, legal stuff, or car mechanics and I have no clue. I hire help, people who've studied this stuff and are experts at it. They can determine what the problem is and help me fix it. But with food, health, nutrition, and weight loss, women tend to think that they should *know* this stuff.

Why? Who taught you? Chances are no one did and it's likely that the family you grew up in had its food issues. (Don't worry, all families do. More on that later.) When you don't know the facts it's hard to create change for yourself. And, in a $70 billion diet industry that's been built on false claims and myths, there's a lot of bad information out there. It's extremely easy to overeat. We live in a society where junk food and fast food are available on every city corner block. But it's also easy to overeat on things that are considered healthy.

My client Valerie was at her wits' end. She was a dietitian, and she was fifty-five pounds overweight. She felt like a fraud in her industry. Here she was, counseling patients on how to get healthy, improve their nutrition, and lose weight, and she was fat. She knew how bad diets were, so she tried other popular methods for weight loss like eating all organic food, she cut out gluten from her life, limited her saturated fat intake, and decreased her meat consumption but her weight didn't budge.

The straw that broke her was when she was working with an obese eighteen-year-old girl who wanted band surgery and her doctor sent her to Valerie for nutrition counseling. This angry, frustrated, young woman sat through her session with Valerie, glaring at her. Finally, near the end, this girl said to her, "I get that you're trying to help me, but why should I listen to you? You're fat like me. What do you know, anyway?"

As I listened to Valerie explain her situation, I could feel her frustration. She kept saying to me that she was doing all the "right" things, but nothing worked. She told me how she had a healthy green smoothie every morning with a whole avocado in it, fruit, yogurt, and juice. Then she snacked on whole, unroasted almonds during the day. At lunch, she said it was typical to have a quinoa salad with black beans and a protein, then she'd snack on more nuts in the afternoon and then have a healthy dinner. After dinner, she'd maybe have some coconut milk ice cream or if she was "snacky," she'd eat gluten-free crackers and cheese. She drank organic wine on the weekends.

Here was this beautiful, smart woman who'd gone to school to help others be healthy, and she was a victim to so much of the misinformation that's out there in the weight loss world. Valerie was simply overeating for her kitty cat body size. Although she wasn't eating "junk," she was eating more calories than she required, so her body was storing all of that excess energy as fat. Once we normalized her eating for her height, age, weight, and physical activity level, Valerie lost weight. She didn't diet to do this. She just committed to slow, steady, consistent weight loss, and she's never regained a pound.

There are two huge areas where your lack of nutrition knowledge is hurting you – it's when you engage in mindless munching and your "witching hours."

Mindless Munching During Your Witching Hours

How many times have you reached your hand into a bag of chips only to realize that there are just crumbs left in the bottom? Or you ate something while watching TV or working at your desk and then looked at the plate and didn't even realize you'd finished it? So often we're putting things into our mouths and we're not even aware of it. This can lead to a huge increase in the number of calories that you're eating in a day and completely halt weight loss from happening. And, worse, it simply becomes a habit.

Mindless munching happens when you zone out. It's a perfect distraction technique. It gives you something to do without having to do anything at all.

The second biggest reason you overeat is to help you cope with things in your life that are hard. You may have a clue what some of those things are or you may be oblivious to some of them. Wherever you're experiencing a lack of something in your life you will use food to fill the void. But you may not even realize you're doing this.

I talk a lot about The Witching Hours. These are the times in your day that you feel the most out of sync and will use food or a glass of wine (or three) to make it through. It could be the mid-morning slump around 10 a.m. or the afternoon crash between 3 and 5 p.m. For most women though, the hardest hours of the day are between 8 and 11 p.m.

This is when you eat even though you're not hungry. You simply *feel like something to eat.*

You will be set free from your weight loss struggles when you start to reconnect to your body and understand when you're truly physiologically hungry and when you're eating for emotional reasons. When you can find the midpoint for your body so that you no longer have to oscillate between undereating and overeating everything will change for you. Your weight, your energy level, your health, your confidence, your radiance, your sense of freedom with food and your body.

To stop overeating, you must start to understand what you're truly hungry for.

True Physiological Hunger versus Emotional Hunger

I'm a big fan of helping women learn how to lose weight healthily because when you do it like that, the weight stays off for good. When you engage in quick and dirty weight loss tactics (like dieting and constantly swinging between undereating and overeating) you'll find the weight comes right back on again. Quick weight loss leads to quick weight regain.

Losing weight in a healthy way requires getting reconnected with your body and being able to identify what it is telling you. It also requires you to pay attention to your emotional self. To do this you must start to discern the difference between:

1. Physiological Hunger

   The sensation experienced in your body when you need to eat food. Typically, you will experience hunger pains around two and a half to three and a half hours after eating your last complete meal.

2. Emotional Hunger

   Using food to satisfy or to deny/distract yourself from what you are feeling (anger, boredom, sadness, and loneliness). It's eating "comfort food" (cookies, chips, ice cream, or candy) even when your stomach isn't growling. It's also known as emotional eating. Understanding emotional eating is important as many women "eat their feelings" without even knowing it.

Seventy-five percent of overeating is caused by emotions, so dealing with emotions appropriately is important.

Five Simple Ways to Tell the Difference Between Emotional and Physical Hunger

1. Emotional hunger will have you scavenging your pantry and fridge because you feel like something to eat – you crave something specific like chocolate or peanut butter or chips. When you are physiologically hungry, you are

much more open to different food options and they are usually healthier.

2. When you are emotionally hungry, you will keep eating well past the point of feeling full. You'll say things like, "I'm full but can't stop eating," or "I know I should stop but I can't." When you eat because you're physiologically hungry, you'll stop when you're full.

3. Emotional hunger can come on rapidly and is generally accompanied by a feeling of "I need to eat X, Y, or Z now (a glass of wine, French fries, cookies) – you'll even drive to go get it. Physical hunger will occur gradually – you'll know that you're starting to feel hungry but if you're busy it can wait.

4. You feel guilty after emotional eating. After eating for physiological reasons, you feel good because your body needed food.

5. Emotional eating is accompanied by an "out of control" feeling – physiological eating is accompanied by calm, in-control feelings.

When I was at my heaviest, I had no clue that I was an emotional eater. I didn't identify with those words. It didn't look to me like what I thought an emotional eater was, which was someone going to the store and filling their cart with chips, cookies, chocolate bars, and ice cream and then coming home and eating it all. That is a form of emotional eating but that's called Binge Eating Disorder (BED) and I didn't have that. Instead, I had something that over the years I had learned to justify and rationalize and it was using food as treats, rewards, and comfort.

To me, I simply liked having a glass of red wine at the end of the day. I like chocolate so it was fun to eat it. And chances are if I wasn't overeating during the rest of the day and consuming high-calorie drinks like lattes and snacks from Starbucks or drinking fruit smoothies from the local smoothie bar, and if I'd stuck to just one glass of wine at night and one tablespoon of chocolate chips, maybe things would have been different for me. As it was, one glass of wine could lead certainly lead to two (sometimes three glasses) and I'd go back to the cupboard two or three times grabbing just a little handful of chocolate chips. I distinctly remember an evening where I'd just finished eating my second handful of chocolate chips and I was holding a glass of shiraz in my hand when I said, "I just don't know why I can't lose the weight. I mean, I'm walking every day." *Groan.*

Hindsight is amazing, isn't it? What I know now that I didn't way back then is that food and wine had become an emotional crutch for me. I'll talk more about this later, but I truly was not willing or ready to accept that my marriage was falling apart, that I was living life feeling lonely and unsupported. I know now that by admitting what was going on would have made me feel terrified as I had dreams of what my family life looked like and I was determined to hang on to my nuclear family and give my children what I never got.

It's sometimes easier to stay in denial because once you admit something to yourself, you can't unknow it. I used food and wine to stay in denial until I just couldn't take it anymore. If you're reading this, then you're at a place in your life where you're being asked to pay attention.

Phew. That was a lot of information. I say over and over again that there are two key parts to a weight-loss journey. The first is understanding the physiological factors that are at play with metabolism and food choices, which was what this chapter was all about. The second key component is understanding the psychological factors that contribute to your success or self-sabotage, which we're about to dive deep into in chapter 6.

6

Self-Sabotage Is Part of the Process

"If you don't change it, you're choosing it."
—Unknown

Okay. This is where we go deeper. Have you ever wanted something so badly, for so long, and you try so hard but you just keep failing? How about losing weight and keeping it off, for example? It can seem so crazy to have this conscious desire (weight loss) and then to consciously do things that prevent what you want from happening (tell yourself that you don't care, say "screw it," and go on an eating binge). It's called self-sabotage and it's 100 percent a part of the weight-loss journey. This chapter will explain exactly what self-sabotage looks like and will give you a six-part framework for helping you stay committed to your heart of heart's desires.

Most women think that if they want something that they'd never do anything to sabotage getting it. Think again. Self-sabotage often exists in our lives because of a lack of self-esteem, self-worth, self-confidence and self-belief. If you don't think you can lose weight or if you've failed at losing weight and keeping it off in the past, then you'll engage in sabotaging behaviors, often without even realizing it.

Yesterday, I got a text message from a friend of mine, Kim, who is extremely self-aware. She said, "I need to lose weight in a fast and healthy way, can you help me?"

I responded, "That's like saying oil and water should mix and they simply don't – fast and healthy weight loss is an oxymoron."

She replied, "Well, I've done it before. I dropped 10 pounds in two weeks in a fast and healthy way, so I know I can do it again. I just always seem to self-sabotage and the weight comes right back on again. I just need a new plan."

Do you see what's going on here? Kim is still chasing weight loss because the way she went about creating that initial weight loss for herself didn't allow the weight loss to be permanent. And, she's dealing with something that all women deal with – not allowing herself to be successful due to the insidious ways she sabotages herself.

There are a million tactics out there that will help you lose weight, and some of them even are healthy.

Here are some of the biggest tips out there on the internet for weight loss. All you need to do is this to see the pounds go (chances are you already know these things):

- Cut out sugar and flour from your diet
- Eliminate all junk food and as much processed food as you can
- Stop drinking alcohol
- Don't eat out
- Get three balanced meals a day and only eat a healthy snack if you're hungry
- Drink two liters of water a day
- Get three to five workouts a week that are of moderate intensity

- Strength train twice a week
- Eat enough protein and fiber
- Meditate, write in your journal, or do yoga as a way to manage your stress

If you want to lose weight in the most efficient way possible, that's all you have to do. You can stop reading this book right now and go off and do this.

Except what happens? Life gets busy, you get stressed out and tired, a fun social event comes up or it's the holidays, you travel for work or a vacation or you simply have a crappy day and "fall off the wagon." And then you stay off of it for months (or years). Until you get desperate to lose weight again and become willing to do anything.

All of the above weight loss tips are included in many of the "diets," "weight loss programs," and "detoxes and cleanses" that are out there. But what I want you to be able to do is create a lifestyle that you can live with knowing that you have the freedom to eat and drink whatever you want, whenever you want, just like I do *and* stay at your desired, ideal weight because you now know *how* to do that. Weight loss or weight maintenance is no longer a mystery.

And that means you need to understand that self-sabotage is part of the process.

The Merriam-Webster Dictionary defines self-sabotage as "the act of destroying or damaging something deliberately so that it does not work." The MacMillan Dictionary says self-sabotage is "deliberately stopping someone from achieving something or to deliberately prevent a plan or process from being successful." Self-sabotage can look like many things but what I see the most with weight loss are behaviors like procrastination, justified excuse-making, rationalizations based on why you can or can't do something, cheating with food, lying to yourself, acting out of integrity – you say one thing and then do another.

When you embark on a true, permanent weight-loss journey, what you're saying is that you're willing to truly change your life. You're willing to change your way of being, of thinking, and your behaviors to create the change you want in your life.

Diets simply ask you to white-knuckle a program for a few weeks.

Sure, the weight will come off, but the minute you engage in self-sabotage and stop following the program, the weight will come right back on again. Hence, the yo-yo diet phenomenon. And that is what creates the emotional exhaustion and frustration with yourself.

You need to know that people would rather die than change. That statement was said to me back in 1993 during my Health Promotion class. I thought it was a bit of an overstatement like you might right now. But think about it…

Do you floss your teeth?

Take a multivitamin every day?

Get your 10,000 steps in?

Eat veggies?

Meditate regularly?

Do you do any of the efficient weight loss suggestions you already know you should do?

Nope. You don't. If you did, you wouldn't be reading this.

When you decide to change your life, you will experience an enormous amount of resistance. Many books have been specifically written on this subject, such as *The Big Leap* by Gay Hendricks and almost everything that was written by Wayne Dyer or any guru in the personal development industry.

The biggest roadblock you face is you and your fear. Very early in my weight loss process, I teach my clients about the Cycle of Change because when you have a context or a framework to lean into, it's way easier to not personalize it

Cycle of Change

Vision

To get to where you want to go, you have to know where that is. It seems simple enough, but do you have a clear vision? Do you know exactly how much weight you want to lose? Do you understand *why* losing weight is important to you? Are you 100 percent committed to this vision no matter what?

For many of my clients, having a vision for weight loss seems dumb or unnecessary. I'm going to assume you own a car, or have been in a car, that works perfectly well and can get you where you want to go. Let's say you get into that car and your goal is to get someplace better than where you're at. You don't know where you want to go. Can you get there?

The car works perfectly. But you still have to get *in* the car and then direct it. Chances are that you've driven somewhere today or you're going to go somewhere. How do you get to where you want to go? You need to know the destination. If you simply got in the car and started driving, it could be frustrating. Even though the car works, you're not getting to your destination.

I recently held a retreat. Clients drove from other cities and flew in from other countries to attend. If I simply told them that the retreat was in the Rocky Mountains and I couldn't wait to see them, would it matter that they wanted to be there? No.

For my clients to get there, they needed to know it was in a beautiful little town called Canmore. They also needed to know the hotel, and more than that, they needed the specific room number we'd be meeting in. Knowing that travel can be tiring and there can be travel delays and detours, they also needed to know why it was going to be worth it to them to make the trip.

If they didn't believe they could get there, would they have even tried? If they had expected to get lost or sidetracked would they even bother getting in the car or on a plane that day? If any of these clients expected to fail, they probably would have just stayed in the comfort of their home.

This is exactly where weight loss goes wrong for most women. You don't have a clear vision of what you want and why you want it. You may have already experienced a setback or roadblock and now you expect your failure. You're far more likely to give up than be successful. You inwardly complain about the journey – you hate that it's so hard, takes so long, isn't fun, and so forth. You will argue more for why you're going to fail than succeed and you start to believe yourself. Your vision lacks enthusiasm and excitement. Without a compelling vision, it's like you're driving aimlessly around, trying to do the right things but not getting anywhere.

Create your compelling vision now. Get out your journal and answer these questions:

1. Who am I when I'm at my best? How do I feel in my body? What's different about it?

2. What will be different for me in my life after I've achieved this?

3. What matters most about doing this for myself?

4. What is required of me to be successful?

You see, often weight loss becomes the all-encompassing life thing that you put your energy into as a way to distract yourself from the other problems you've got in life. By answering these questions you're forced to come to terms with why this is important to you and for your life.

Here is how my client, Sierra, answered these questions:

> "When I'm at my best I'm confident, strong, and feel happy. Life feels easier. I laugh more. I feel more at ease. There's a peacefulness in my heart instead of all of this anxiety that I feel. I feel sexy in my own skin, desirable… I'm no longer trying to hide myself or not be seen. It's like I emerge from the shadows into the sun. Honestly, it's like I feel like "me again." What's different in my life is that I'm going after the things that I want… I no longer feel invisible or like I'm not good enough. I feel capable and powerful. The self-doubt is gone and instead I feel self-assured. I know who I am and I like myself. My husband likes me too – we've reconnected. I've brought that confidence back into our relationship and it's made a huge difference in our ability to be intimate. I'm more loving, not as defensive or snippy with him… I don't take everything as a personal dig like I used to. I'm a better parent too. I know I'm a good role model because I'm healthy – inside and out. It's so important for me to be a good example to my daughters – I don't want them to struggle the way I have. In order for me to be successful? Geez… I need to believe I'm capable of change. I need to be kinder to myself and believe in myself. I have to let go of the negative voice in my head. Honestly, I need to truly go after it… not just make a half-assed attempt like I usually do. I need to believe it matters because it does… this is my life. I deserve these things. I deserve to feel good."

Decision

After your vision is clear, you have the next important step to take. You have to decide if you're going to go after it or not. Once you lay it on the line and take stock of why this life change is important to you, you now need to put the frontal lobe of your brain to work and make a solid, conscious decision. You may have many different visions in your life and each one will require your energy.

For so many women, trying to lose weight is like an afterthought. It's like this, "I'm super busy with work and the kids, and I need to make my deadlines and blah, blah, blah, and then if I have enough energy leftover, I'll take care of myself." And then you don't. This is why you're at the weight you're at.

Many women live in the land of ambiguity. They say they want something but do nothing about it, or just barely do enough to pretend that they're trying, which allows them to feel better about themselves. This is why ten-day cleanses are popular.

This may be the worst place of all to be. It's like one foot in, one foot out. You're at the beach. A few of your friends have run splashing into the waves and are having fun, completely in the experience of it. Then you've got another group of friends who are lying on their beach towel, relaxing and soaking up the sun. They decided to *not* go in the water.

And then there's you. You're walking along the shoreline with one foot in the water and one foot out. You're looking to your friends in the water having fun and back at your friends on the beach relaxing and you're trying to decide what to do. You're miserable. You can't decide. Each decision makes you think you're going to be missing out or that it's going to cost you something or you're worried you're going to make the wrong decision. You waffle going back and forth with what you want to do. Because you're completely stalled out, you refuse to make a decision.

If you refuse to decide, you're refusing to take charge of your life and change. It's that simple. Think back to the last time you started a diet because a friend asked you to do it with her or when you felt so tired but simply needed to try something to help you lose weight. Was it successful? No.

It's time for you to decide what you want. You do have choices available to you. No one is making you lose weight. You can either accept yourself at the weight you're at and no longer give it power in your life, or you make a decision to go on a weight-loss journey and accept the challenges that come with the journey, holding onto the deep conviction that it's worth it.

I never tell clients what weight they should be. It's a personal decision. For some who've been in the 220s or more, being under 200 pounds would be a dream come true. They literally would be ecstatic to see 190-something on the scale. For others, they've reached a number they've never seen on the scale (maybe it's 170, 180, or 190 pounds) and it's a wakeup call. For others, it's losing the baby weight they gained and never lost, and fitting back into their favorite pair of jeans again. For my clients who are 300 pounds or more, it's about choosing life, they know that their weight is a risk factor for illness, and they want to live.

What I don't abide by is women being told that they should simply give up and accept the body they're in. This doesn't make me a popular voice in the body-positivity crowd. My message gets confused. Be body positive *and* do what it requires for you to create change for yourself. Don't succumb to self-sabotage or bad information or crappy diets and allow that to be the reason you fail for good. For my clients who've tried this approach, just accepting themselves as they are after they've tried to lose weight and have failed makes them feel hopeless. They've been told things by their doctor or other health professional like:

- It's your hormones
- Weight loss is way harder after forty
- You're weight loss resistant
- Your medications all have weight gain as a side effect

I fundamentally believe that women should have the knowledge and support they need to get to their destination. These are two critical elements that are neglected in most weight loss programs. They stay at the superficial level and typically don't give women the lifestyle tools and strategies or healthy belief systems that they need to be successful in the long term.

For women who've tried accepting themselves overweight, they do this with disappointment, resignation, bitterness, and resentment. I hear comments like:

- I just don't feel like me
- My outside doesn't match my inside
- I don't know who I am like this
- I just don't feel right; this isn't how I'm supposed to live the rest of my life
- This can't be it

Eventually, they'll try another diet.

I said or thought all of those same things when I was at my heaviest. The real reason it didn't feel right to be at that weight was that I was harming myself with food and using it as an emotional crutch. I lacked some basic understanding of food, fat metabolism, and weight loss, and that made me feel frustrated. I engaged in self-sabotage because I didn't fully understand the Cycle of Change that I'm teaching to you now.

On the flip side, you cannot hate yourself thin. There's no amount of self-loathing, self-hatred, or self-deprecation that's going to motivate you to create true change in your life. It just makes you feel horrible about yourself. Fact: you've already tried this. I know the voice in your head all too well. It's the voice all women have. It's the voice of "you're not enough." It's not true. But when you start with a compelling vision and fully step into making a life-changing decision for yourself, love is required.

Take out your pen and paper again and make a decision about what you're going to do, write it down. Don't write down what you're *not* going to do, that doesn't work as well. Instead, focus on where you're going.

Action

Deciding without taking any action is simply wishing or hoping for something to happen. Nothing changes until you change it. This means you've got to take a step forward that cements your decision.

I have a friend, Sarah, who decided to do her PhD. She made that "decision" ten years ago and she still hasn't started. She never took any action on her decision. She has a million reasons (i.e., excuses) as to why she's waited. An action step for Sarah would have been to review PhD programs and then apply to the top programs that she wanted to be accepted into. And, not surprisingly, Sarah's weight hasn't changed either. She's still carrying an extra forty pounds on her body and talks a lot about doing something about it, but never does. Making a decision but not taking any action allows Sarah to pretend that she's trying and moving forward in her life but in all honestly, she's just staying stuck in her comfort zone.

It's the same with my client, Candice. Candice started running marathons and half-marathons in her early twenties. She loved it. Her dream was to lose weight and get back into running shape. She came to one of our coaching calls in the winter and joyfully told me that she had decided to do it – she was going to do a ten-kilometer race in the spring. She made the decision but never signed up for a race. Needless to say, she didn't do it, she didn't run in a race.

In the spring, Candice said she'd decided to do a race in the fall and explained that spring just hadn't been the right time for her.

Making a decision is important. Following it up with an action step cements your commitment to your vision.

This is the third part of the model. Taking action. Action is important because it shows the universe and the world around you that you're serious. It's a declaration that you're willing to expend the energy to change rather than the emotional energy to stay stuck. I wasn't about to let Candice make a decision without her locking it in with action. Her homework was to review the races she was interested in and email me her race registration confirmation by Friday.

The minute you take an action step often huge chaos will erupt in your life. It may be that you get sick or perhaps you get transferred to a new city or a parent becomes ill. This can leave you feeling like you're on the verge of a breakdown, and this is where *many* women will go, "Oh, it's obviously not the right time for me to do this right now," and then quit and justify why they've quit, which is due to the life storm/chaos. Instead, I want you to know that this is normal, and you are to view it as a test. It's a test of your commitment. It's like the Universe is asking if you want this or are you going to be easily swayed and stop.

Predictably enough, this happened to Candice, too. She emailed late on Thursday night explaining that one of her kids had been sick and she hadn't had a chance to research races. She told me that she had to work late on Friday as her boss was on vacation and now she wasn't sure if she could do this. I quickly replied that I expected to see her race registration within twenty-four hours.

Candice emailed me the next day and followed it up with a quick phone call. "Jen. I did it. I'm registered. I'm so excited and scared and I realized that's why I didn't sign up in the spring – my fear about whether or not I could do this was holding me back so I just didn't take any action. It all makes sense now, I was stopping myself before I even let myself start so I didn't have to deal with disappointing myself... ugh. Crazy, isn't it?"

No, it's normal.

The other beautiful thing about taking action is that it creates confidence. Most people want to wait until they feel confident to go out and do something, but it doesn't work that way. Confidence doesn't just land in your lap. It's created. The only way you can create confidence is by taking action. The action step is what will allow you to experience a win, it may be a tiny win, but at least it's a win and that's what fuels your motivation. Do you notice how when you feel motivated you take bold action? The more motivated you are the more actions you take, the bigger your wins get. The wins allow you to feel successful and that success builds your confidence.

Candice ran that ten kilometers and now three years later, she's completed her seventh marathon. She's changed jobs, increased her salary by 20 percent, and started internet dating after being single for five years. How did she do all of this? She got her confidence back.

For weight loss to happen, you have to take action. You can't sit back and wait or meditate your way to a healthier body. The more committed and consistent you are with your actions, the bigger your wins (i.e., the loss on the scale). If you want something to change in your life, you have to change it. If you get clear on your vision, make a decision and take action, change is inevitable.

Fear

It's time to call a spade a spade. The biggest barrier to creating change in your life is fear. This doesn't mean that you walk around all day feeling fearful. It's not like that. Fear is sneaky. It can show up as procrastinating, engaging in self-doubt, being skeptical and cynical about the likelihood of succeeding, listening to the mean voice inside your head, and simply not feeling like doing it.

Fear is your mind's way of keeping you stuck. It tries to trick you and make you believe your excuses and limiting beliefs. If you've been a chronic dieter and have years or decades of negative belief systems stacked up about who you are or what's possible for you then you better believe the fear of failure is getting in your way. The accumulated disappointment over the years of trying and failing to lose weight leaves an emotional scar. Only you can see it. The idea of losing weight has become so distant for you because it's been so disappointing in the past, and you may be afraid to try and fail again. Who wants to keep trying at something and failing? It's like banging your head against a brick wall until its bloody. It hurts. It can seem easier to just not bother. Especially when it seems like you need to get more extreme with each weight loss method you try – eventually, it's just not worth it.

Or you might be like my client Sam who discovered she was fearful of being successful with her weight loss. She said to me, "I just don't know what I'd be like or who I'll be as a thin person." It sounds so strange but this happens a lot and there are good reasons why. For Sam, she and her friends used to make fun of the "skinny chicks" that they knew. They would get together and pick on them behind their "thin" friends' backs. Sam was afraid that if she lost weight, all of a sudden, her friends would turn on her because she'd now be one of the "skinny chicks." Sam was also afraid of the new freedoms and possibilities she'd have in her life. Her weight had always been her legitimate reason for holding herself back from going after things that she wanted in her life – if she no longer had that excuse, what if she went after something and didn't get it?

My client Ali was secretly afraid of losing weight for two reasons (she didn't know these reasons even existed for her until we did a coaching call and dug a little deeper). When Ali was nineteen and in college, she was date-raped. She was terrified that by losing weight, she would receive all sorts of unwanted attention from men, and she didn't know how to handle that. Further, Ali was also in a mediocre marriage. Before we started working together, she asked me, "How many of your clients leave their husbands in this process?" It was a curious question.

What was also interesting was that her husband kept saying that she was going to get all "hot and confident" and leave him. When you take the action steps to achieve something that you didn't think was possible, you truly do become a different person. Your confidence will skyrocket. You'll have renewed faith in yourself. You'll have new dreams for your life. And sometimes that does mean leaving people behind you. But that's not a bad thing. It can just feel scary.

Here's the real thing about losing weight, you're choosing to create change in your life. Change is uncomfortable. Many people in your life may not want you to change. They like you just the way you are and so they'll try to keep you there (more on that later). Plus, if being overweight has been your primary reason to live a small life and you are no longer overweight, you've lost your primary excuse. It forces your hand.

How fear can get in the way of weight loss:

- It may cause you to face things about yourself or your life that you don't want to face
- You don't know who you will be at a different weight, you're stripping away your identity as the "chubby," "fat," "happy," or "fun" girl
- You don't know how to handle unwanted attention
- You're afraid you might lose friends or change the status of your relationship
- You'll leave things behind that no longer serve you and you're afraid of hurting people

When you truly get clear that you are 100 percent committed to losing weight and you desire to stop using food to numb your pain or distract you from the hard things that are happening in your life, everything can feel raw, exposed, bare, tender. You can feel like you're going to "snap," or like you can't handle it, can't cope, and that's normal. You've essentially stripped away the security blanket and now you're choosing to face what food/booze has numbed for you. This is exactly why you must commit to a new vision; create a new story of possibility for yourself.

What I want you to do the next time you feel fear coming on, while you're in the process of making a change in your life, is to say, "Ha, sneaky fear. I was expecting you. You don't get to stop me this time," and then lean into taking action and getting support.

Cheerleaders

Anybody who's ever done something amazing has not done it on their own. They have support: a team of people working with them, a coach for direction and leadership. And cheerleaders.

Seriously, think about this. Politicians have speaking coaches and a whole team of advisors. Athletes have coaches, personal trainers, massage therapists, sports psychologists, and fans. Musicians have their vocal coaches, talent agent, publicists, and their fans. The top CEOs in the world have mentors, business coaches, strategic advisors, the board of directors, and so on.

Who do you have in your corner?

Most of the women I know give and give and give all day long. They give to their families, their boss, their clients, and the dog. They give their energy outward, and how do they replenish? They don't. They are exhausted. Perhaps you are exhausted too.

The *biggest* myth in the weight loss world is that *I can and should be able to do this on my own.*

Aye yai yai. It drives me crazy. Why? Why does this exist?

If you need a cavity filled, you go to a dentist. If you need surgery, you get a surgeon to do it. If your car needs fixing, you go to a mechanic. Why? Because you *trust* that they're going to get the job done and do it right. They are experts.

You need to create a group of cheerleaders when it comes to weight loss. And, of course, I recommend you get a weight loss coach; they know what they're doing. They can help you get the job done and make it easier. But aside from that, you need people around you who believe in you and who share your enthusiasm for your vision. They need to pick you up when you are down and celebrate the wins along the way with you. Isolation is the enemy of weight loss success. The go-it-alone method is a recipe for failure.

The sad thing is that sometimes our cheerleaders are not who we want them to be. The people closest to you may be the ones who sabotage your efforts the most. It's crazy, but true. Why does this happen? The people who love you just want you to stay safe and be happy. They don't want to see you hurting or disappointed.

They have unconditional love for you and sometimes they want you to do what they're doing too so they have company.

When I'm up to something big in my life, like writing this book, I never tell my mom at the beginning. She worries and frets and tells me that I'm taking on too much and that I just need to take it easy. How is it going to affect the kids and am I sure I can write a book? Her fear jumps up to the forefront and it can trigger *my* fear. All of a sudden, my excitement, enthusiasm, and confidence has turned into self-doubt:

- Oh no. Maybe it is too much, can I take this on right now? Is this a dumb idea?
- I don't know if I can write a book; I think I suck at writing, maybe my mom is right.
- It's going to take too much time. Maybe I should do this later when I'm less busy.

Do you see how crazy-making that is? What you need when you go after something big in your life is for people to be excited with you and have the ability to hold your vision for you when you get discouraged or tired. That's what cheerleaders are supposed to do.

Think of any sports team that was down and out and losing. Did the actual cheerleaders just decide to sit on the floor and not cheer? Did they say to the team, "There's no point, you're losing?" Or did they cheer even harder for their team? That's right. They cheered harder. They pour their belief, faith, and confidence into their routines to help remind the players that they can win. I want you to play to win at weight loss so go write down who's going to be on your cheerleader team. Pick three to five people who are going to support you, encourage you, and expect your success. Have a conversation with each of them and tell them exactly what support looks like for you. Often people don't know how to give you the support you need. The last thing you want is for one of your cheerleaders to be like, "Hey, it's okay you've had a bad day. Let's go get some ice cream. That will help you feel better." No, no, no!

Celebrate

Most successful women I know accomplishment-hop. They go from one success to another while barely taking a breath. They'll often pretend that what they just did was no big deal. I've seen this from my CEOs who did successful company mergers, to women who cooked a beautiful dinner and then said it was nothing. Sometimes they even nit-pick and share all of the things that went wrong instead of celebrating what went right.

This happens all the time with weight loss. You crap on your successes and wish things were better, faster. You get angry and feel upset that you lost only a pound and think it should've been more like three pounds. The problem with this is if you don't celebrate your wins, then you're only focusing on your failures and the weight-loss journey becomes exhausting. When it gets too exhausting, you'll quit.

Instead, I want you to celebrate every single win. I want you to be proud of every healthier choice you make and feel elated with yourself when you say "no" to something that you would have said "yes" to before. Be grateful that your clothes are getting looser. Feel excited that you have more energy during the day. Be proud that the mean voice in your head is getting quieter. These are the wins that diets don't tell you to focus on. And give yourself a high-ten in the mirror for every pound that comes off your body because that took your effort, faith, commitment, and persistence. In the weight loss world we call these NSV's – Non-Scale Victories because it's not just about the number you see on the scale. That's just one data point and there are so many other things to be proud of.

Let's sum this up: the Cycle of Change involves six critical steps: vision, decision, action, fear, cheerleaders, and celebrate. There are times when I'm moving through these steps and reminding myself of them every hour. I literally can work this cycle many times in a day. Life happens. You can't lose weight in a bubble because you don't live your life in a bubble. Instead, you need to know the framework of what's involved with change and work it, baby.

The Thing That Hurts My Heart the Most

Lastly, the most insidious thing attacking women right now is the epidemic of "Not Enough." I hear it over and over again, and I've experienced it myself. This is when self-doubt and limiting beliefs have accrued in such a way that you can't see your brilliance or magnificence anymore. Instead, your mind plagues you with all of the ways you're not enough:

- Not thin enough
- Not sexy enough
- Not smart enough
- Not pretty enough
- Not ambitious enough
- Not brave enough
- Not talented enough
- Not good enough
- Not fit enough
- Not funny enough
- Not poised enough
- Not confident enough

I could go on and on with this list, but I won't because it doesn't serve anyone. When we engage in the "not enough" conversation, it's like swimming in a toxic soup. It can make you feel sick. The only person who can change this conversation in your head is you. It begins by asking yourself how thinking these things are helping you.

The short answer is, they're not. You're harming yourself and holding yourself back from your life. Something you have to understand is your thoughts generate your feelings which influence your actions which create the outcomes you experience in life.

Thoughts → Feelings → Actions → Outcomes

If you don't like how something is in your life, then it's time to go back and examine your thoughts because you can change those. You have complete sovereignty over your thoughts. You are the one who chooses them. You're the one who allows your thoughts to rule you.

When you think something negative, it's common to feel crappy and it's typical to take lousy actions and then you get the negative outcome.

→ Thought: I'm not disciplined enough to lose weight
→ Feelings: Unhappy, scared, unmotivated, angry, bitter, resentful, et cetera
→ Actions: Go eat a bag of chips, ice cream, chocolate (because what's the point?)
→ Outcome: Stay the same weight or gain weight

When you get truly ready to change your weight, it will start with how you think about yourself, your abilities and the weight-loss journey itself that will have the highest degree of influence on your success.

It's so easy to get stuck at a particular step in the Cycle of Change or in the isolation of the "not enough" conversation because it's become your habit to do so. Procrastinating is a habit. Choosing to not make a decision is habit. Self-neglect is a habit. Taking start-stop action and chasing Mondays is a habit which is why I'm so excited for you to read chapter 7. Understanding why you do the things you do and how to create change in your life is all about understanding your habits.

7

Hunger, Hanger, and Habits

"She remembered who she was, and the game changed."
—Lalah Deliah

I came across Charles Duhigg's book *The Power of Habit* when it first came out and devoured it one night. I tried to learn everything I could about why we do the things we do. Reading that book changed my life and has allowed me to change hundreds of women's lives when it comes to food. I discovered exactly why diets feel so depriving and why women can only white-knuckle them for a certain amount of time.

Here are some basic facts about habits. First of all, you are the sum of your habits. The things you do every single day have created the reality/world that you live in. You can change your habits. That means you can change. What's interesting is learning why you do the things that you do.

Habit Creation

Habits don't just come into our lives out of thin air, they are developed by making conscious decisions. The outcome of that decision either makes us feel good or bad. If it makes us feel good, then we'll do it again. Before we know it, we no longer are consciously thinking about what we're doing, we just simply do it.

For me, nine years ago, at the end of a long day, I poured myself a glass of red wine and grabbed a handful of chocolate chips. As I was reading Charles's book, I started to ask myself why I used to do that. When did I start doing that? It was something that I did without thinking about it and now I was trying to dissect what was going on for me. What I learned was fascinating.

Charles explains that there are three parts to the habit loop: the cue (trigger), the routine (the habit), and the reward (what you get from doing what you're doing).

The Cue

Let's talk about the first part of the habit loop: the cue (or the "trigger). There are all sorts of things that are triggers in your life:

- A certain time of day (I call these your witching hours)
  - 10 a.m. – first break of the day
  - 3 p.m. – stressed about completing your work on time
  - 5 p.m. – driving home, have tons to do that night
  - 7 p.m. – driving kids around to their activities
  - 10 p.m. – house is quiet; you have some alone time

- People (annoying boss, your spouse, your kids, your colleagues, your mom)
- A feeling state (sad, irritated, bored, lonely)
- A place (the kitchen, the office break room, the TV room, Starbucks)
- Thoughts (could be negative or positive)
- An event or occasion (holiday parties, family get-togethers)
- A preceding event – what just happened?

Here's the thing about cues: they're nearly impossible to get rid of. You live in a world that functions with the twenty-four-hour clock. You're going to encounter 3 p.m. every single day for the rest of your life. Chances are that you're not going to cut out or disconnect from all of the people in your life who trigger you. You're human, so you're going to continue to have a range of emotional experiences. You're going to encounter the same spaces; you can't just go live in a bunker. Your mind has 80,000 thoughts a day. Holiday parties and weekends and family get-togethers are going to happen for the rest of your life. So, you can't just delete the cues in your life.

It's normal to develop a routine to cope with the cues in your life and it becomes almost instinctive over time, it becomes your habit. And we attach a lot of things to our habits – we judge them, critique them, feel either good or bad about them. But few people understand the role of habits in their life. And ultimately the quality of your life is based on the quality of your habits.

The healthier your habits are, the healthier you'll be. It makes sense, so why do we create habits that don't help us or make us happier? You can look at your habits in any area of your life:

- Parenting – are you a yeller or a calm talker?
- Money – are you a spender or a saver?
- Fitness – are you a couch potato or daily exerciser?

I'm going to stick with looking at your habits around food since food is what contributes to 95 percent of weight loss issues.

The Routine (Habit)

The routine refers to the thing that you do in response to the cue. You can look at this for any aspect of your life but I'm going to be focusing on your eating habits.

What are some of the things you eat when you are exposed

to one of your triggers? I ask this question every time I teach a live workshop and the answers are always the same:

- Cookies
- Crackers
- Chips
- Chocolate
- Brownies
- Nuts
- Candy
- Popcorn
- Cheese
- French fries
- Pizza
- Ice cream
- Nachos
- Wine/beer/cocktails
- Marshmallows

Now, what's interesting is the third part of the habit loop. Understanding this is what changed everything for me and typically for my clients too which means I'm sure it'll be a lightbulb moment for you.

The Reward

I used to think that I just drank wine and ate chocolate because I liked it. I have clients who say the same thing, "But I just love ice cream, Jen. That's why I eat it." And, if we left it right here, then it would make sense that if you simply stopped eating the ice cream you'd lose weight, right? Why is it so hard to give up something you like? Is it just because you like it?

No. You get an emotional reward out of eating the thing that you like.

The third part of the habit loop is "The Reward." Rewards are powerful and often they are subconsciously driving your behavior. This is why it's not enough to simply tell yourself you're not going to eat something – it's because you crave the reward that eating the particular thing gives you.

Let's talk about some of the most common rewards that hundreds of women have identified when we dug a little deeper into the questions of why do we do what we do, and what is it that you're craving?

What does eating/drinking your favorite things give you?

Here's what women have said – "Eating or drinking gives me..."

- A break
- A chance to escape my reality
- The ability to numb myself
- To forget about it
- A moment of peace
- Distraction
- A way to feel happy
- Something to do
- Felt calmer
- A sense of fun
- Belonging
- Love
- Companionship
- Didn't have to think or worry about anything

What's imperative to understand here is you don't just eat the cookie or the chips or the chocolate or drink the wine because it tastes good, you do it to fulfill an emotional need or want in your life that you're craving to be fulfilled. Our emotional cravings become representative of our food cravings.

Whatever is lacking emotionally in your life, food will fill the void. And food is easy. You can always count on food. It's always there. It doesn't expect anything from you, it doesn't talk back, it doesn't fight with you or tell you what's wrong with you. It's simply there, available 24/7 for you.

This is the real reason diets fail you (notice how I didn't say you fail at dieting?). A typical diet tells you to get rid of all of the foods you are currently relying on as your emotional crutch. Except you may not have seen it that way before. Diets tell you to simply use willpower, commitment, and discipline and ignore your food cravings. Except eating these foods *has been* the way that you've fed yourself emotionally. Now, when you cut out the food it also means that you don't get any of the emotional rewards in your life that you're (sub)consciously desiring. This is why dieting feels so depriving. There's a soul hunger that exists deep within you and junk food has been the way you've fed it.

This is why diets suck. This is why they don't work. This is why we have to change the conversation around what it takes to lose weight and keep it off. We have to disrupt the dieting culture. It's not as simple as "eat less, move more." It's about creating a life that you love and fulfills you. It's about creating and maintaining healthy boundaries. It's about no longer tolerating what isn't working in your life and taking action to course correct those things instead. It means having hard conversations – with yourself and others.

Focusing on simply eliminating the foods you eat that have contributed to your weight loss troubles is a narrow solution that doesn't work in the long run. This is why you may have lost weight in the past but put it right back on again.

Meal plans, work out plans, eliminating food groups, restricting the times that you eat are all surface-level tactics designed to give you the short win. The long win comes when you recognize why you're overeating in the first place. Something is missing in your life and you're using food to fill the void. That may be painful to acknowledge and you might want to go eat candy right now, but it's the truth.

You Can't Change What You're Not Aware Of

If you haven't been aware of the true emotional needs that you're longing to have fulfilled, you can't change. The first step is awareness. If you choose to stay numb in your life, thinking it's better to avoid than deal, you will stay overweight. True change requires a deep understanding of what's going on for you emotionally and physiologically.

When I reflect on my life ten years ago, I see a young woman who felt completely alone in her marriage and was exhausted by having a baby and a two-year-old while trying to start a company. She was isolated, unsupported, and scared. But all of that was too much to admit. She denied the reality of what was going on in her life and she ate chocolate and drank wine to have moments of relief.

I have hundreds of stories like this one. Stories of women being bored at night so they ate. Women who worked in jobs that they couldn't stand so they ate. Women who were married (or single) and were lonely and didn't know how to change it. Women who were saddened and exhausted by looking after a sick and dying parent, so they ate. Women who had lost their dreams and forgotten their worth, so they ate. Women who were once powerful, confident beings and they became lost and insecure, so they ate.

Then they hate themselves because of their weight. They shame and blame themselves and criticize themselves for having no control or will power. They do what the dieting industry tells them to do, they diet to try and lose weight.

And they fail. Over and over again. With each failure, they lose themselves just a little bit more until the pain becomes almost crippling. It's a vicious cycle because they want to avoid the pain and disappointment they feel in themselves so they eat more. Their weight increases while their self-esteem plummets.

It's time for the craziness of being on the dieting hamster wheel to stop. And the only way to do that is to become aware of your deepest truths and your darkest fears. It's time to take responsibility and get clear on what you truly need and want in life and to go after it.

It's time to change your habits but to do so, you have to recognize and understand why you're doing what you're doing, for real. Not with the dieting spin put on things.

Thoughts and Feelings as Habits

So much focus in the dieting world is put on what you *do* as opposed to what you think. But your way of thinking can be a habit and as just discussed in the previous chapter:

Thoughts → Feelings → Actions → Outcomes.

So, if you have habitual thoughts that go unchecked or that you're not even aware of, then you're creating possible outcomes for yourself that are way easier to change than you even know. That's fantastic news. Simply becoming aware of your thoughts gives you the chance to ask yourself, "What am I getting from thinking this? What's my emotional reward?"

Truly, for many women, thinking that they aren't enough on any level, allows them to stay safe. They might not like it, but at least it's familiar.

Let's go back to *habits* for a moment and summarize a few key things:

1. You most likely will not be able to eliminate all of the cues/triggers in your life – you will be able to change some of them (thoughts/feelings) but others will remain the same (twenty-four-hour clock, your kids will stay your kids, et cetera)

2. You are a human being who has emotional needs; it's impossible to give up on having those emotional needs met

3. The current routine/habit you have of meeting those emotional needs isn't working for you because it's preventing weight loss from happening (in some cases, you're even gaining weight)

4. It's time to experiment with non-food-based ways to get your emotional rewards met

Here's how Charles Duhigg explains how to change a habit. First, he says you have to identify your routine, the exact behavior you want to change. Then you have to determine the rewards that you're getting from doing what you're doing. Lastly, you can piece together all of the triggers that exist for you that cause the habit to happen.

When I look back at my weight-loss sabotaging habits of drinking wine and eating chocolate I work through the framework like this:

1. I want to stop drinking wine and eating chocolate on a nightly basis

2. The rewards I'm getting are an escape, distraction, a treat, and a moment of joy

3. I engage in this habit typically between seven to eight p.m., once I've put the kids to bed, the house is quiet, I'm alone with my then-husband, I'm in the kitchen

There are a lot of triggers in that situation. The fourth step of changing a habit is to experiment with giving yourself other routines to engage in that will still give you the reward you're trying to get. The different habits I experimented with were taking a bath, going out for a walk, making tea, and doing something creative with my hands. Now, in the beginning, *none* of these were as satisfying as drinking wine and eating chocolate. But I wanted to lose weight so I was willing to experiment and see what worked. In the end, making a cup of tea became my new go-to nightly habit. I could now trust that even with all of those cues/triggers in my life, I could make tea, get some of my emotional needs met and lose weight.

Pro-weight loss tip – stop telling yourself what you are *not* going to do, and instead tell yourself what you *are* going to do. The brain hears these messages differently. If you tell yourself, "I'm not going to drink wine tonight," your brain hears "I'm going to drink wine tonight." Whatever you tell yourself that you can't have, you end up wanting it more. Instead, tell yourself what you are going to do: "I'm going to make tea tonight and enjoy it."

"I'm not going to miss any of my workouts this week" becomes "I'm going to do all of my workouts this week."

"I'm not eating any junk food today" becomes "I'm going to eat healthy, nourishing food today."

Diets are typically cheap, fast, and easy. You focus on surface-level stuff and create temporary surface-level change. Eventually, you get frustrated with this crazy-making yo-yo diet, weight gain, weight loss cycle and you know you need to do it differently which is why you're reading this.

True change is exactly the opposite of dieting. It requires the investment of your time and energy, it requires long-term effort but the good news is almost any habit can be reshaped. And if you remember the first sentence in this chapter, it said, you are the sum of your habits, so if your habits can be reshaped, so can you.

So much of the diet rhetoric out there says that you just need to have more willpower and discipline to be successful with weight loss, but you already know I don't believe that. I like to make things as easy as possible for myself and that means not trying to white-knuckle my way through change. Instead I focus on creating an environment around me that supports the change I'm creating. Let me show you how to do just that in the next chapter.

8

Plan, Expect, and Create Your Success

"My dreams are not here to make you comfortable."
– Unknown

Many women have been told that they just need to have more willpower and discipline to lose weight. This is an ineffective statement at best and psychologically harmful at worst. Like a muscle that fatigues over time, so does willpower and discipline. When women lose their ability to hold or maintain their willpower and discipline, they start to think of themselves as a failure or like something's wrong with them. This is simply not true. Let's talk about some easier things that can be done to support yourself along your weight-loss journey. The first is learning how to set your environment up for your success.

I don't remember where I read this but I remember feeling awestruck by this simple statement – it was something like this: "We are all on a see-food diet, if we see it we eat it *and* you can't eat what you don't see." A lightbulb went off in my head. What if I could create systems and strategies for my clients where they didn't have to rely on willpower and discipline and instead made all of this simple for them? That's what this chapter is all about.

I want to share these practical strategies with you so that the minute you're done with this chapter, you can go and take action. I want you to experience success while you're reading this book. I promise we'll get to the deeper emotional issues too, but this will allow you to experience some wins right away.

Change Your Environment to Support Yourself

Changing things up in your kitchen is probably the easiest place to start. Think about it – when you're tired or feel hungry, you probably walk into your kitchen and the first thing you do is scan your countertop. Then you open up your pantry and the first thing you see is what is at eye level. Often, what's on the shelves at eye level are things like crackers, chips, cookies, granola bars, and cereal. That's what you'll choose to have. If you open up your fridge, perhaps you see things like cheese, leftover desserts, or that bottle of white wine, and all of a sudden you feel like having that. It's critical to shake up things in your environment so those aren't the first things you see. Here's how to do that.

Kitchen Makeover

It's time to move food around in your kitchen. Specifically, it's about putting food away so you can't see it. If can't see it, you won't be as likely to eat it. Let's start with your countertop.

Kitchen Counter:

- Clear off your kitchen counter so that there's nothing on it. Get rid of the clutter. This includes paper clutter as well. The clutter we see creates clutter in our minds. This means no cereal boxes, loaves of bread, crackers, cookies, baked goods, bottles of wine, hard alcohol, pop bottles, et cetera – put it all away.

- The only things allowed on your counter are a water pitcher, a fruit and veggie bowl, and a blender.
  - o The fruit bowl can have lemons, limes, apples, tomatoes, and one to two other choices of your favorite fruits.
  - o Put away any containers/bags that contain treats.
  - o If there's a toaster on your counter, put that away (people with toasters on their counter are more likely to weigh ten to twenty pounds more than people who don't have a toaster on their counter).

- Give your counters a thorough cleaning – it makes it nice and tidy and feels like a fresh start.

Remember, visible foods are the ones you'll eat first. Let's tackle the second major problem area: the pantry. It's easy to tell yourself that you're not going to eat something and that you're going to make healthier choices, but add a little stress into your day or if you're feeling a little tired, it's pretty easy to grab the chocolate or the cookies if you see them. Let's change up your pantry so the healthy choices are the ones you see first.

Kitchen Pantry and Cupboards:
- Throw out any nearly empty package – let's make some space.
- Throw out anything stale or outdated.
- Make sure all boxes/bags/jars/containers are sealed so that there's no easy access as you breeze by (I call this being "bag lazy" or "lid lazy" – it was one of my major challenges with chocolate chips).
- Make your tempting treats/foods inconvenient to get to.

- Put them up high in a cupboard or on a shelf in your pantry so you can't get to them (need a stool).
- Put them into a storage bin with a lid (not see-through) and store them down low or at the back of a cupboard.
- Remove them from the cupboard/pantry altogether – put those items in a storage container and place it downstairs, in your garage, or storage closet.
- This includes items that you know are trigger foods for you or are "go-to" comfort food – this may include chips, crackers, chocolate chips, chocolate bars, candy, packaged cookies, breakfast cereals, granola bars, dried fruit, pop, and juice.
- If you store your alcohol in the pantry, put it in a box or storage container with the lid closed. If it's in a cupboard, push everything to the back so you can't see it when you open the cupboard.

Fridge

Once you've done your counters and pantry, you've done 80 percent of the work. All that's left now is your fridge and freezer. I want you to take *everything* out of your fridge and give it a good cleaning. Before you do your next grocery shop, take an hour or so and follow these tips and recommendations. They may sound strange at first and not at all how you're currently doing things so these changes may make you feel uncomfortable. I say, "Fantastic." But just think back over the past week or month and ask yourself how many rotten, gooey vegetables have you thrown out lately. If you're like a lot of my clients, you go to the store, buy your vegetables, put them into the drawers at the bottom of the fridge, and forget about them. When you see them rotting, you pull them out, throw them away, and go and buy new ones. There's a better way.

Strategies for a healthier fridge:

- Throw out any condiments that are old or you just never use.
- Stop using your "crisper" drawers for fruits and veggies – instead, fill those with other things. (Make one a meat/cheese drawer, use another for any less healthy snacks or leftover desserts. I use one of our drawers for condiments.)
- Put your vegetables and fruits on the middle shelves that are at eye level. Store them in clear storage containers or bags – arrange it so that's the first thing you see when you open your fridge.
- Put your healthiest snacks on the main, eye-level shelves: Greek yogurt, cottage cheese, hummus, guacamole, pre-cut veggies.
- Wrap any of your "treats" in tinfoil – for some reason, this just works.
- Take out any pop or "energy drinks."
- Empty any juice cartons you had (or finish them, but don't replace them), and keep a pitcher of water in the fridge instead (you could also just put that on the counter).

The last place to do a quick makeover of is your freezer.

Freezer

Don't underestimate the power of your freezer when it comes to getting healthy and cutting back on snacks. Here are a few handy tips to make your freezer work for you:

- Throw out anything that has freezer burn on it
- Have frozen veggies in it – peas, corn, and green beans are my favorite
- Have one to two frozen bags of berries or other pre-cut fruit

- Great place to keep nuts and seeds fresh so they don't go rancid

What's the point of all of this?

We're changing it up, so things are "out of sight, out of mind." This means that you can't just walk into your pantry and grab that bag of candy. You have to truly think about it and want it to go get it. This works and doesn't rely on you thinking you need to deprive yourself or use your willpower to not have something. No willpower or discipline is required if you haven't even seen something because then you don't have to tell yourself that you don't want it or can't have it. We're tricking your brain.

As stated before, you are a creature of habit and if left to your own devices you'll go back to your old ways, so changing your environment is critical to changing your habits. Having a fresh, well-organized fridge/freezer and pantry is such a treat – plus, you eat what you see and now you're only going to be seeing healthy things.

The Four Ps

You can do all of the emotional work you want, but if you don't have practical strategies to rely on, then weight loss can feel like a lot of work. When you choose to remain in health or nutrition chaos then weight loss simply can't happen. There's an element of feeling in control of the day and the week and when you are, then you're not leaving your weight loss up to "chance" or hoping that you'll lose weight this week. You know that you've set yourself up for success.

Plan

Life is busy and if you're not making a plan on how to be successful with your weight loss goals then you're (sub)consciously planning to fail. That's a hard truth. You've got to become pro-active instead of reactive in regard to the meals you're going to eat and the type of food you're going to consume. Here's what "Planning" looks like for me and what I highly suggest it should look like for you:

Plan the days that grocery shopping will be done (typically two days a week) and put that in your calendar

Plan when veggie prep is going to happen (usually need two sessions of about thirty minutes)

Review all of the activities for the week and determine how many nights you're out of the house and when you need to eat dinner by

Plan at least one day a month to do some batch cooking to help with those busy nights

Plan out your grocery lists ahead of time and make copies of it so you aren't always starting from scratch

Meal Plan

Meal planning can feel daunting at first but think of all the other things you give your time and attention to and create a plan for. You probably spend time planning vacations or parties. You probably have to create plans at work or to get things done in your day. A plan gives you a roadmap. A critical element of weight loss is creating a meal plan for the week. I know, I know… groan, right? "What's for dinner?" is the question I used to hate the most, especially when it was asked at 5 p.m. and I didn't know the answer. Often, that leads to getting pizza or grabbing takeout from somewhere because I simply didn't have the time or energy to run to the store to grab groceries. You have to take the time to plan your meals for the week. This is a key step to being successful in shifting to long-term healthy lifestyle behaviors. Start with just writing out your dinners for the week. Write down what protein you're going to cook and what veggies you plan to have. Skip to the Thank You page in this book to find out how to get one of my meal plan templates.

Purchase

You can have the best laid out plan in the world but if you don't get to the grocery store and stock your fridge and pantry with healthy foods, nothing can happen. Now you have to go get your groceries but you've already determined which days you're going to do that on so it's no longer an "after work surprise or chore." Before you do that, create your grocery list from your meal plan for the week and add anything else you may need for simple breakfasts or lunches. Stick to the outer edges of the grocery store – only go into a middle aisle if something is on your list. Avoid the bulk section as well as the chip/cracker/pop/candy aisles. Purchasing "fresh" is great but frozen works just as well.

Prepare

This is another critical step and one that most women don't take. Once you get home with that load of groceries, don't just throw them into your fridge to be forgotten about. Get out your glass storage containers and dedicate an hour of your time to doing all of your veggie prep. This includes washing, peeling, chopping, slicing, dicing, and grating.

- Wash: everything (lettuce included)
- Peel: carrots
- Slice: celery, carrots
- Chop: broccoli, cauliflower
- Grate: carrots, beets, cabbage

98

This one little tip can be a lifesaver on busy days and nights. Salads become instantly easier to put together because everything is already done.

Pack

If you want to lose weight, you can't rely on eating out to help you with your weight-loss journey. You'll eat lion-sized portions, and restaurant food is always packed with more oil than home-cooked food. Invest in good Tupperware or glass storage containers. From this point on, you will always pack food so that you're prepared and not caught out and about "hungry." This includes packing your lunch and packing food/snacks on weekend days.

The Golden Rules

I don't provide my clients with many hard rules around food. What I ask them to pay attention to is how much they're having (the portion), of what (the type of food/booze), and how often they're eating it (the frequency). It's been almost nine years since I went on my weight-loss journey, and I now eat and drink whatever I want, whenever I want. I have complete freedom with my food choices and my weight has stayed the same for nine years. It feels so easy, and, yes, it can be easy for you. But I do follow these five golden rules. They provide simple do's and don'ts that help me take better care of myself and don't require me to use willpower or discipline.

Sit Down When You Eat

It seems basic, but think of how many times you "grab and go" or eat while standing up or rushing around. Give yourself the gift of time when you eat. Think of how you used to feed your toddler – you sat your child in a highchair, smiled, interacted with, and fed your son or daughter one bite of food at a time. You waited until they swallowed and then you provided another bite of food. There was no rushing. Give yourself this kind of love and patience with meals.

Don't Combine Eating With Any Other Activity

Often eating gets combined with another activity like watching TV, working at your desk, scrolling through your phone, answering emails, and so forth. This is the easiest way to engage in mindless eating where you're not even conscious of what you're putting in your mouth or how much. You are completely disconnected from nourishing your body and you're often not getting any pleasure from the experience. The rule is if you're going to eat, then sit down at a table or countertop and eat, but don't do anything else. Give yourself your attention.

Portion Everything Onto a Plate or Into a Bowl

The days of eating out of a bag or a box have come to an end. The reason for this is simple – it's impossible to know how much you're eating of something and human beings aren't wired with a shut-off switch in their brain. Often, you simply eat until the bag is empty which is typically way beyond what the recommended serving size of the item was. Think back to the last bag of chips you had or a king-sized chocolate bar. This was my client Mary's problem. She always intended to "just have a few chips" or just three squares of chocolate, but she almost always ate the whole thing because it was simply there. This kind of overeating leads to being overweight. A simple strategy is to put what you want on a plate or in a bowl and then put the box/bag away.

Eat Slowly and Chew Your Food Thoroughly

If your habit is to rush through life because you always feel so busy, then you may be rushing through the act of eating and barely chewing your food (or tasting it). *Slow down.* If you tend to shovel food in and eat quickly, you won't give yourself the chance to feel your body's hunger and satiety cues. Most of my clients say they eat till they're full or well past full, but they don't know it and can't stop in time. It takes time for your body to register how much food you're putting into your body. Digestion begins in your mouth. Chewing your food thoroughly allows for your digestive enzymes to be secreted which helps with digestion. When you rush this process, it can often lead to feeling bloated.

Don't Eat in Your Car

No discussion, no debate – just follow this rule. I talk a lot about being a creature of habit and eating in the car can be one of the worst habits if you're trying to lose weight. Why? Think about it – when was the last time you ate something healthy in your car? I've heard so many stories around this – stopping to get gas on the way home and you see the two-for-one chocolate bar special so you think to yourself, "That's a good deal, I need that." You go into pay for your gas and grab a couple of chocolate bars and/or a bag of chips because there's a "bonus" deal on. Or you're taking your typical route home from work past your favorite fast food spot and you all of sudden find yourself at the drive-through window ordering onion rings just because.

You might be thinking, "But Jen, this sounds like so much work." You're right – going on any journey requires that you take the action to get prepared so you can get to your destination. And you need to take this action whether you feel like it or not.

Let me put it to you like this: think about the last vacation destination that you flew to. You didn't just teleport there, did you? No, there's some work to be done ahead of time. Things like finding the best airplane ticket price, doing research to find the hotel you want to stay at, planning out any trips that you might do and booking them, going shopping to get whatever clothes you or your family may need. Then you need to get to the airport and check-in.

You can do *all* of that work but you're still not at the destination yet, right? You have to get on the plane. And when you're on the plane, you don't quite have the same freedoms as you do on land but you're okay with it because eventually, you know you're going to be able to get off the plane and be at your destination. This is *exactly* like going on a weight-loss journey. You can do all sorts of pre-work, but if you don't get on the plane, you're not going to get to your destination. Sometimes your flight plan can have layovers or it may not be a direct route. Sometimes the plane is turbulent. Being on the plane is not quite as comfortable as being at home. What would happen if you were on the plane and then opened the door to get off? Well, you most certainly wouldn't get to your destination, would you? Most of my clients do lots of "pre-work" for weight loss: they think about it, take some action, but they never get on the plane, so to speak. If they do get on the plane, often, they want off of it. They open the door and step out, and then they free-fall back into old habits. This is called self-sabotage, but more on that later.

What I want you to understand is that you have to recognize that you're going on a journey. It's a journey that will have some unexpected ups and downs, but it's worth it to get to your destination – *permanent weight loss*. A weight-loss journey can feel uncomfortable in the beginning because you can't keep doing what you're doing and get a different result. Things have to change. *You* have to change.

Stop Letting the Scale Ruin Your Day

Back when I was overweight, I would weigh myself around ten times a day. That's about seventy times a week, and each time the number that would show up on the scale had incredible power over me. It could make or break me emotionally. My guess is that you can relate to this.

I want you to understand what the scale is telling you. Unlike a lot of weight loss coaches out there, I don't believe in getting rid of your scale. Neither does the weight loss research. What numerous studies have shown is that weighing yourself once or twice a week is considered a "weight loss best practice," as it's necessary to track changes over time. What I don't believe in is letting the scale ruin your day or fling you into a bout of depression due to the number on it. The scale just gives you data. It's letting you know if what you're doing is working or not so you have the opportunity to course-correct.

There is a right and wrong way to use the scale. The wrong way is to do what I used to do. I'd get up, go pee, and stand on the scale. Then I'd move the scale to a different location to see if I'd get a different number. I'd get on and off it three or four times and then I'd look at my naked body in the mirror and direct hatred toward what I saw reflected. I'd feel frustrated and gross and confused. How could the number be up when I tried so hard and was so good yesterday? Ugh.

Then I'd get dressed, have breakfast, do a few things, and then go poop. I'd immediately get naked and go stand on the scale, thinking that must have made a difference. Nope. I'd repeat this process throughout the day, before exercise, after I'd exercised, before dinner, and the worst one of all would be before bed. I'd stand on that scale, see the number on it, and then go lie in bed wrapped in a feeling of self-loathing. I felt disgusted by my body. I'd put my hands on my belly, squeeze my fat, and hate myself. It was horrible.

This is the embarrassing part – as you know, I have a master's degree in exercise physiology, and I just didn't understand why I had these wild fluctuations on the scale. I mean honestly, I could gain five pounds in a few hours when I'd hardly eaten a thing. How was that even possible? Not understanding how to interpret the scale data created stress, anxiety, frustration, and toxic thoughts about myself.

So, let me set you straight on what the scale is telling and how you can make peace with it so it no longer hijacks your emotions and makes you feel like a failure.

Understanding body composition is critical to understanding healthy weight loss. Body composition is a term used to describe the different elements that make up your body. Your body is made up of:

- Muscle: ranges from 30 to 50 percent of your total weight
- Bone: about 15 percent
- Fat: less than 10 percent (exceptionally lean) to greater than 50 percent (morbidly obese)
- Water (blood): ranges between 50 and 65 percent, varies from person to person

As an adult, your bone weight is not going to change much and when you're on a healthy weight-loss journey the goal is to preserve as much of your muscle mass as you can. That leaves the other two components, fat mass, and body water. When you stand on the scale you only get a composite number of these four elements – you have no idea what is causing the changes and the word that automatically pops into a woman's mind is thinking that she's gaining or losing fat.

But that's not the whole story.

Daily weight fluctuation is normal. The average adult woman's weight fluctuates up to four or six pounds per day and this is due to body water fluctuation, not the gain/loss of fat mass. You see, one liter of water weighs 2.2 pounds and it's normal to experience body water fluctuations between one to 2.5 liters a day (that's 2.2 to 5.5 pounds). Water weight is different than fat weight, but I guarantee you that when you see that number go up you don't think to yourself, "Hm, I wonder if that's due to my intracellular water fluctuation today?" You think, "Ugh, what is *wrong* with me? I just gained five pounds." And, then you think, "Screw it, I'm just going to go eat a bag of chips and a tub of ice cream anyway because no matter what I do nothing works."

You can see how weighing yourself multiple times a day can make you feel like a crazy woman; all you're doing is seeing the scale number fluctuate due to normal body water fluctuations but it makes you feel like a failure. The truth is that you're not.

Now you might be wondering, "Why does water weight go up and down like that?" Great question. There are a few things that cause water weight to increase:

1. Eating salty foods (think restaurant food or if you add a lot of salt to your meals)
   Hormonal changes during the days leading up to your menstrual cycle (this gives that feeling of being bloated)
   Eating a large number of carbohydrates; for every gram of carbohydrates stored in the body as glycogen, you retain two-to-three grams of water

Let's talk about point number three here for a moment. If you've ever done Atkins, tried eating a paleo diet, or gone keto, you may have noticed that during the first week you were on this diet the scale reflected a significant drop in weight. I've had clients tell me that they've lost ten pounds in one week but then they get so frustrated after in the weeks to come when the rate of weight loss slows.

The reason so much weight is lost in the first week or so isn't that you've dropped ten pounds of fat, you simply have shed a significant amount of body water due to no longer eating carbohydrates. Alternatively, I've had women say that every time they even look at a slice of bread, they gain five pounds. *But* we're not talking gains or losses of fat. We're talking about the body doing its job to either store or release carbohydrate and to do so it either has to retain or release water.

Makes sense, right? Sure, when you understand the chemistry of the body and how food interacts with it. But most women don't know this. they simply feel like they're an emotional slave to the scale and it gets them down.

Let's talk about the right way to use the scale.

Best Practices for Using the Scale as a Healthy Tool

Stop weighing yourself every day.

Instead, weigh yourself once a week (at most twice) on the same day and time – record your naked scale weight and focus on eating more healthy choices and less junk.

It's just a number – don't let the scale make or break you emotionally.

Always remember why you're doing what you're doing and hang on to the bigger picture. Sometimes seeing the number go "up" can create a sense of panic or depression along with thoughts like "Why bother?" or "There's no point." This can lead to self-soothing with food and hijack your weight loss goals.

Seeing the number on the scale drop can make you want to celebrate – have an extra glass of wine, eat the dessert, or have second helpings. Don't do it. Stay committed to the process and you'll reach your goal.

Don't let the scale be the only judge of your weight loss efforts. Take stock of how your clothes fit. How much energy do you have during the day? How do you feel? The scale is simply one data point. When you get hyper-focused on it, you can lose sight of all the other incredible changes you're realizing.

What you have to understand is that to lose weight, you have to give your body the correct signals to burn fat. That takes both consistency and time.

Think about it like this: have you ever been to a bonfire? What happens when a log of wood is put on the fire? Does it combust and turn into ash immediately? No, it takes time to burn. That's exactly like fat. Fat is like a log, and you have to create the fire-like conditions in your body for it to be metabolized and used as fuel. This is why you need to give yourself time to see fat loss happen. And that doesn't happen hour-to-hour or even in a day. This is exactly why consistency is so important in a weight-loss journey and how being "good" three or four days but then falling off the wagon for a few days takes you right back to starting over and chasing Mondays. No more of that.

I get that this chapter is kind of all the typical stuff you might already "know" but don't do. And that's what the rest of the book is about. closing the gap between what you know and what you do so you can have lifetime success with weight loss.

By now you might be wondering where exercise fits in with all of this? One only needs to scroll Instagram to see all of the hardcore workouts out there that are promising life-changing weight loss results. But have you noticed that most of those Instagram fitness celebs are young, nubile twenty-somethings who have no difficulty contorting themselves into a pretzel on the floor while doing a one-finger push up in a weird yoga pose? An exaggeration? Perhaps, but it holds some truth as well and I'm about to share the truth with you regarding weight loss and exercise.

9

You Can't Out-Run Your Fork

"Strong women don't have attitudes. They
have standards and boundaries."
—Rahul

I'm going to set the record straight on a few things here: exercise is amazing for you for a million reasons but weight loss isn't one of them. That's right. If you're trying to use exercise as your method to lose weight, then you are going to fail because you will never have enough hours in the day to out-train an unhealthy diet. What you stuff into your face during a ten-minute emotional eating episode or after three hours of watching TV and engaging in mindless munching (chips, popcorn, nuts, etc.) could take you four hours to exercise off. Who has time for that? When women come to me telling me all of the different ways they've tried to lose weight, exercise is often is at the top of the list and they're exhausted.

When I carried my excess thirty-five-plus pounds and felt miserable, I didn't understand a few things. You see, although I ate well most of the time (my main meals, at least), I ate like a lion. Add on the "extras" and the glasses of wine during a week, and I consumed more calories than my body needed. I didn't realize this. I had the idea that I ate "well" or "healthy," so food couldn't possibly be the problem. I was sure the problem was that I didn't exercise enough and that when I did, I'd lose weight.

Now, this can screw women two-fold because if you're like me and love to exercise, then you look forward to it and ultimately start to hate it because it's not getting you the results you want. You push harder, longer, feel frustrated, and then start to give up. And if you're like a lot of my clients, you may hate exercise and believe that your weight loss problem is going to exist for the rest of your life because you simply don't like to exercise.

Here's the good news. The days of punishing yourself on a treadmill or having to dress in skintight eighties aerobic gear and sweat it out for an hour are over. The amount of research that has been done on physical activity and health indicators in the past fifty years is staggering.

But let's start with the basics.

Diet and exercise are both important factors to pay attention to for good health. By diet, I mean the food you put in your mouth, not the current fad weight loss diet that's out there. What you put in your mouth has a much stronger effect on weight loss than exercise does, yet being a regular exerciser has a strong effect in preventing weight regain after weight loss and assists with weight maintenance.

This was astonishing news to me. As someone who spent her twenties running marathons and doing triathlons, I never paid attention to the food/energy balance equation. I didn't need to. But as a mom with two young kids who were busy I didn't have as much time to exercise, and as a woman who was engaging in emotional eating without knowing it, I had to figure out what exactly was going on.

Here's the challenge: when you rely on exercise as a weight-loss tool, you're leaving weight loss up to chance. Why? Because when life gets busy or the kids get sick or you do or you have pressing deadlines at work or you're traveling, what's often the first thing to go from your schedule? That's right: exercise. There are even more excuses and barriers to exercise, such as thinking things like:

- I don't have time
- I don't want everyone to watch me at the gym, I don't know what I'm doing
- I'm injured
- I hate running
- I hate classes
- I hate doing weights
- I'm too tired
- I don't like wearing tight exercise clothes
- I want to go to classes, but I don't want to be the fat one; I'm embarrassed
- I get discouraged because of how much I've let myself go, trying to exercise just reminds me of that
- I'll go to a class or the gym once I get in shape

The truth is, what you don't feel comfortable or competent at, you'll avoid. It's pretty easy to find a justifiable reason to avoid exercising.

When I committed to getting back into shape simply because I wanted to feel strong and healthy again, I wore loose black pants, an oversized cotton t-shirt, and a ball cap. I remember the first time I walked into the gym. My cheeks burned because I felt so embarrassed and I was sure people were looking at me, wondering why I was even there. I didn't make eye contact with a soul. Having been a personal trainer, it felt so strange to feel this way. The gym used to be like my second home. I was so ashamed that I'd let myself get so out of shape. It was something that I was in denial about, and going to the gym required me to face the truth. I was sure that everyone in the gym was silently laughing at me – the fat loser who didn't know what she was doing. I lasted about ten minutes that first "workout" and then left with hot tears streaming down my face.

The real truth was that no one was paying attention to me. Everyone in the gym was focused on their workout and they were all busy doing their own thing. I went back to the gym the next day. You see, I had a vision, and I'd made a promise to myself to get back in shape, so I kept that commitment. Slowly but surely, week by week, month by month, my body started to change. What once felt so difficult, I could now do easily. Here's the lesson: if you want something to change, then you need to be the one to change. Thinking, wishing, wanting, and hoping doesn't count for much if you don't take any action.

So how come exercise doesn't work for weight loss?

The "move more, eat less" equation is outdated. The truth is that when you move more, you need to eat a little bit more, but that's not what typically happens. Exercisers tend to overeat, which does one of two things. It either prevents weight loss from happening or you will gain weight when you start an exercise program. I've even heard my clients tell me that they must be gaining muscle after a week of exercise because the scale has gone up. Um… no, you're not.

Here's what's happening:

- You typically overestimate how many calories you burn during a workout and so you allow yourself more "cheats" during the day.
- It's common to "reward" yourself with food for being "good" after doing your workout. I can't tell you how many times

I've seen people go to Starbucks after being at the gym and order a latte and a slice of lemon loaf – in that ten-minute snack, they've consumed more than they burned off in the one hour they were at the gym.

- Exercise can stimulate your appetite, although this is believed to be psychologically influenced as research indicates that exercise is an appetite suppressant.
- You will unintentionally take bigger portions on the days you exercise.
- Your trainer or the latest magazine article says that you should eat something before/during or after your workout, which leads to the consumption of unnecessary calories (they'll often recommend eating a bar or having a high-calorie drink of some sort).

All of this can lead to weight loss purgatory. You work super hard but don't see any changes (sometimes it can even lead to weight gain).

Unless you live under a rock, you know that exercise needs to become a part of your lifestyle for the health benefits which extend far beyond weight management. We now know that regular physical activity can help reduce your risk for several diseases and health conditions and improve your overall quality of life. Here are some of the benefits:

- Decrease your risk of heart disease and stroke
- Lower your blood pressure
- Raise your good cholesterol (HDL) levels and lower your bad cholesterol (LDL)
- Improve blood flow and the strength of your heart
- Reduce your risk for Type 2 diabetes or help you better manage your diabetes

- Strengthen your bones and decrease the risk of osteoporosis
- Improve your muscle strength, endurance, and flexibility while decreasing your risk of falls due to poor agility
- Help you better manage stress
- Decrease your risk for depression and anxiety

Quite frankly, I want to be able to have the leg strength to get off the toilet when I'm eighty. I want to be able to *get* to the toilet.

All kidding aside, one of my goals is to be able to be a strong, active woman when I'm eighty years old. I know that how I choose to take care of my body now will have a direct impact on me achieving that goal. I want to live independently for as long as I can, play with my future grandchildren, travel with my husband, and live a life of adventure until the end of my years. This simply can't happen if I engage in self-neglect and don't take care of myself. It can't happen for you either. This is why exercise is important. Not for weight loss, but for overall better quality of life that you get to experience both mentally and physically.

How to Start Exercising Even If You Hate It

The biggest challenge I see for women is that they bring the dieting mentality of "all or nothing" to exercise. It's like there's this myth out there that the only way you can consider yourself an exerciser or get the benefit from it is if you do it for an hour a day, seven days a week and make it intense and hard.

Yuck.

Well, if you think that, no wonder it's hard to get started. That sounds horrible. Instead, I invite you to create a FITT Formula. FITT stands for frequency, intensity, time, and type. Here's the best way to get started.

Step 1: Type of Exercise

Start by brainstorming any type of exercise you either used to enjoy or have been curious about trying. It could be things like Zumba, spin classes, swimming, a bodyweight class, running, kickboxing, and so forth. There are so many boutique fitness studios now there is truly something for everyone. The reason you're starting with picking the kind of exercise you want to do is that if you hate something, you won't do it. Those sneaky excuses will come rocketing back in and you'll stop yourself before you even give yourself the chance to start. Eventually, you will want to incorporate both aerobic and strength training sessions into your week but start with something you enjoy, then build from there.

I had a client named Mallory. She *hated* running and would constantly tell me about how she was going to start running "soon," or after she lost the next five pounds, or when the weather got nicer. I finally asked her "Mallory, if you hate running so much why do you continue to tell me that you're going to start running?" She paused and then said, "Because I want to lose weight. And running is exactly how my sister stays so fit and healthy so I'm going to do that too." I then asked, "Mallory, does your sister like running?" "Oh, she loves it. She was a track star in high school and went to university on a running scholarship."

"Mallory, I don't want you to run... ever." There was silence on the other end of the phone line. "Why not?" Mallory asked. "Because you hate it, which means you're never going to do it consistently. Your excuses will always win out. Accept it – running just isn't your thing. Let's figure out what is."

There was a long pause and then Mallory burst into hysterical laughter, "I just can't tell you the relief I feel knowing that I don't need to run. It's freeing. I no longer feel this weight on my chest or pressure to spend my time doing something I hate. It just felt so hard to get going but I kept telling myself that's what I needed to do." I told Mallory that I understood and it was a common myth that running was a good weight loss strategy. I asked her to write down all of the activities she used to enjoy or think she might enjoy and then pick four to five activities/classes this month to try.

Long story short, Mallory went and tried out a bunch of different classes. At the end of it, she fell in love with Orange Theory, a popular heart-rate based interval training class. She loved the group setting, the variety, and there was a studio in her neighbourhood so it was convenient.

The key here is to remember that you are creating a lifestyle for yourself which means you need to enjoy what you're doing. And to be honest with you, I don't always enjoy starting a new fitness routine if I've been inconsistent for a while – it feels hard, as it should – I'm out of shape. My body needs to adapt to the stimulus I'm subjecting it to and that takes time. If I've gotten used to doing nothing, then doing any kind of new physical activity makes my heart rate go up, my breathing rate increases, my muscles begin to ache sooner, and I want to quit. But the only way to get in shape is to start. That's how it gets easier and how you get stronger and healthier.

Step 2: Determine the Frequency

The "go hard or go home" approach is so 1980s. Let's skip that. Instead, consider how many days a week you can fit an exercise session in. Saying that you're going to exercise seven days a week when you're traveling most of the week or have a crazy deadline that you need to meet just isn't going to happen in the beginning. Be realistic. There's no purpose in setting expectations so high that you likely will fail, set yourself up to win instead. Success builds on the feeling of accomplishment, not the feeling of failure.

In a way this is just like the Planning step when it comes to food. Here you're planning out your exercise. For me, planning my exercise looks like this. At the beginning of every month I map out my exercise dates and I do my best to make them non-negotiables in my life. I put them into my calendar and include the travel/change time I might need. Then on Sunday night I review my commitments for the week and make any adjustments I need to ahead of time in order to make the days and week feel smooth. I plan to exercise when I travel for work, am attending workshops or conferences, and even when I am on holidays.

Now, here's the real truth about how this goes for me because it's often easy to think things like, "Oh it's so easy for her. She must always love going to the gym or running or whatever." Honestly, I don't. There are days when I argue with myself all the way to the gym. It's like I have a good angel on one shoulder telling me how great I'm going to feel after my workout and a bad angel on the other shoulder telling me that it's fine for me to blow off this workout, that there are other things that are more important and I can do this later." The bad angel voice is loud and convincing. It makes me feel guilty. It tells me that I should be spending time with my kids or working or doing anything other than taking care of myself.

But what I do have going for me is my commitment to my vision. Even though I can hear that bad angel, I still go. I've made a rule for myself that if after ten minutes of doing my workout, I still want to quit or leave, then I can. That's happened twice. Starting is always the hardest part which is why I love going to things where I have accountability, like classes or a scheduled personal training session. It forces me to keep those exercise dates.

Back to you. Let's look at a few examples of how you could set this up for yourself.

If you've currently been doing nothing, then committing to exercise two or three times a week would be a great start. Pick what days would work best in your life and write those days down. Then, in your calendar or on your phone, make an exercise date with yourself and be committed to keeping this appointment no matter what. Your brain will tell you that it's ok to skip it, or that you'll just bump it to tomorrow. Don't do that. This is where you're focusing on building a lifestyle habit for yourself and taking action is what will get you the long-term win. Starting is the hardest part. Always. The point is to just do it.

If you've been an inconsistent exerciser over the years but in general like exercise and used to be fit, you may consider creating three or four exercise dates in your calendar. The goal here is to take an objective look at your life and plan for your success. The goal is also to go slow. It takes time for your body to adapt to the new physiological stress you're putting it under. Too much exercise too soon can cause injury. Be safe. Go slow. And commit to a routine.

Step 3: Time

Now you need to decide how long you are going to spend exercising. Going from nothing to an hour isn't wise as you risk injury and having it feel so hard it prevents you from wanting to exercise again. Be realistic. Start slow and know as you get more fit you can increase the length of your workout. The good news is that research has proven that even doing ten minutes of exercise a day can create better health outcomes for you so if that's where you need to start, do it. The point is to just do something.

When you are just starting a new exercise program, typically the time is shorter and the intensity is low. This is to allow your body to adapt to the new physiological stresses you're putting on it and not get hurt. Let me share Karen's journey with you. Karen hated exercise. She was a self-declared "couch potato." She said she wasn't good at exercise, didn't like it, didn't feel good doing it so she didn't do it. Except Karen had lost thirty pounds and was interested in doing everything possible to keep the weight off and stay healthy. She joked that she wanted to get off the toilet when she was eighty, too.

Karen cultivated her exercise routine over a period of five months. She started with two walking sessions a week that were fifteen minutes. At first she wasn't sure if she could make it around the block but she did. And she was proud. She then added in a third day of walking. Over the months she increased from fifteen minutes to twenty, to twenty-five, to thirty minutes to eventually an hour. She felt amazing. She felt ready to incorporate some basic bodyweight strength training exercises so we cut her walking back to forty-five minutes per session and she then started doing fifteen minutes of strength training.

Fast forward three years. Karen just sent me a picture of herself after she completed her first half-marathon and she was all smiles. In her email she said that never in a million years would she have *ever* thought she'd be a runner. Karen is fifty-six now and has maintained her weight loss for three years and has no fear of regaining any of it, ever.

Gradual progression is the name of the game here. Something is better than nothing – start with an amount of time for your exercise session that you know you can do and build from that.

Step 4: Intensity

Determining the intensity of your workout is based on your initial fitness level and how much time you're devoting to a workout. Intensity is defined as the amount of effort or work that is invested in a specific exercise workout. It's important to ensure that the intensity is hard enough to overload the body but not so difficult that it results in overtraining, injury, or burnout.

For example, if you already have a decent fitness level and don't have a lot of time, higher intensity workouts will typically provide more benefits (such as burning more calories in a shorter amount of time). For example, choosing to jog (more intense) may require only thirty minutes of commitment versus walking (less intense) which may require forty-five to sixty minutes.

I often see women starting to get back into exercise and they go out too hard, for too long, and feel super sore the next day or two or get injured and then they don't want to do it because it sucks feeling this way. Like weight loss, building up your fitness level takes time. It requires patience and a commitment to yourself to show up and do it.

How Much Do I Need to Exercise?

There are all sorts of independent and government-funded national research bodies around the world and they have all created similar guidelines and recommendations which are as follows:

- Aerobic exercise: Do a minimum of two and a half to five hours of moderate aerobic activity a week
- Muscular strength: Engage in two strength training sessions a week that target the main muscle groups of the body

Here are some basic principles to know:

- Anything is better than nothing: even starting with a five-minute routine can help you
- Start now: health benefits can be quickly experienced

- Be physically active throughout your day by taking the stairs more often, parking further away from stores and walking more, play with your kids and grandkids, get outside more often

Will Weights Make Me Bulky?

No. Lifting weights will not make you bulky.

Lifting weights is what shapes and tones your body. In the twenty years I've been in the health and fitness industry, I've had numerous women come to me asking how to tone their bodies. They think cardio is the answer. It's not.

If you want to see your body toned or if you want to take it further and get ripped or shredded, then you have no option but to learn how to strength train properly.

I've been every kind of fit a woman can be. I've been marathon fit, Ironman fit, extremely-ripped-gym fit, fitness class fit, and I've also just been normal healthy fit. I can promise you that your body is incredibly mold-able and shape-able but you have to do the work. When you put in the time and effort, you get the result. Remember all of those barriers to exercise? Yeah, those often get in the way.

When I was marathon fit, I was running five days a week to build up my mileage to over fifty miles a week – that's a lot of hours spent running. When I was Ironman fit, I spent four hours a week in the pool, ten hours a week on a bike, and up to ten hours a week or more running. That's a *lot* of hours spent exercising, but I had a goal so I did the work. When I was super-ripped-gym fit, I spent six hours a week in the gym, lifting heavy weights doing three to five sets of twelve to fifteen reps, and I also got my cardio in. And now, I am healthy, fit woman who follows the same FITT principles that I'm advising you to create. I don't have a specific training goal in mind at the moment, and certainly nothing that's extreme. Normally, I spend about two hours a week in the gym strength training, I walk my St. Bernard puppy about an hour a day, and I do three fitness classes or spin sessions a week for cardio. I do this because it makes me feel good, and, remember, I want to get off the toilet when I'm eighty.

When you want to change your body, you need to be willing to do the work to change it.

All of this helpful info about how to set yourself up for success and bringing the habit of physical activity into your life will result in few real changes to your weight if you don't understand why you're overweight in the first place.

I'm circling back around to what I said at the beginning of this chapter, which is that you will never, ever have enough hours in the day to out-exercise an unhealthy diet. It is way easier to overeat and consume excess energy than it is to burn it off, thanks in part to what we covered in chapter 4 regarding the food companies and how they choose to produce our convenience foods and junk food products.

For instance, drinking a grande caramel macchiato from Starbucks (240 calories) would require you to exercise for thirty minutes on the elliptical machine or to go for a fifty-five-minute walk. If you order a side of fries with your lunch (400 calories), you would need to go to a thirty-minute kickboxing class to burn off those calories. Did you have a slice of pepperoni pizza for dinner? Then you now need to go for a fairly intense run for thirty minutes or so. Getting a bag of chips from the vending machine when you felt snacky? Go hit the gym for an hour to burn off those 240 calories.

And what if you ate all of this in one day? You would need to exercise for around three hours to create energy balance and to not have those excess calories that your little kitty cat body doesn't need to get converted and stored as fat. This isn't a sustainable way to live as you simply don't have time for that.

It's far simpler to understand the nutritional requirements of your body, the energy or the caloric density of the food choices you make, and how to nourish yourself from the inside out for optimal health. This includes understanding why you overeat in the first place.

A common complaint that I hear often is, "Jen, I know better. Why don't I do better? I'm just so frustrated with myself." I get it. I truly do. I've been there and I've coached hundreds of women who felt this way once too. The dieting world has failed women because diets only focus on one part of the equation – the food piece. The other part of that equation is the emotional and social aspects we have in our lives and how being human can just be hard sometimes. Life can be hard sometimes. Let's find a way to allow weight loss to be easier.

10

I Know Better. Why Don't I Do Better?

"I create the rules of the game and I play to win."
—Jennifer Powter

You will hear me say this over and over again: going on a weight-loss journey is the ultimate personal development work. It's a transformative process and women will often personalize it and make up stories about being weak, not disciplined, or having no control. None of that is the truth.

To be successful in permanent weight loss, you have to understand a few components around the psychology of behavior change and what's going on in your brain. Essentially, we need to reprogram your brain for change to happen. It's not just about calories in or calories out. It's about why you eat what you eat in the first place and what's driving that.

When I went through my weight loss transformation I became fascinated with the field of neuroscience – understanding why we do what we do and what drove that behavior. I love research, I love science and I'm a nerd at heart. I've been an avid student of this science for the past ten years and love learning.

Neuroscience is the multidisciplinary branch of biology that combines physiology, anatomy, molecular biology, developmental biology, cytology, mathematical modeling, and psychology to understand the fundamental and emergent properties of neurons and neural circuits. Essentially, studying neuroscience helps create an understanding of the biological basis of learning, memory, behavior, perception, and consciousness. Or, simply put, why you do what you do.

I want you to recognize and deeply understand that what you're engaged in right now isn't just weight loss – you are reprogramming your brain. You are learning how to think new thoughts about yourself and have new neurons wire and fire together. You are unpacking decades worth of neural linkages in your brain. This section is a little science-y but understanding this will bring you some peace of mind and make you feel like you're not failing, instead you're learning a new way to accomplish permanent weight loss.

Conscious thought drives about 5 percent of your behavior. That's not much. Ninety-five percent of your behavior is being driven by your subconscious mind. The subconscious mind has deep imprinting from when you were little. The years zero to nine are the most critical forming years in terms of what we think about ourselves – those years can influence our sense of self, self-esteem, self-efficacy, self-confidence, and self-worth.

So much can happen in those years. Whether you had an amazing childhood or a horrible one, you learned how to survive and how to protect your emotional energy. Your survival instinct is incredibly strong. So is the desire and ability to escape emotional or physical pain. All any human being wants to do is to numb the pain and to try to do something that makes them feel good. Food can make you feel good. So can booze.

Here is how this plays out. Perhaps you pull out a pair of jeans to get dressed one morning and they're tight and you think, "I have got to do something about this." So, a new thought enters your conscious mind: "I'm going to do whatever it takes to lose weight."

But what you might not be aware of is that you've got all of these little thoughts and limiting beliefs running through your subconscious mind. These are things that you think and feel about yourself based on your past experiences. You may not even know some of the things you think about yourself because thinking this way has become your habit, it's your version of "normal" and from this way of thinking you've created rules for yourself.

Look at it this way – life is a game and you're the one who created the rules to play by. When you have a new thought, it's like you're saying that you want to change the rules of the game. And you are going to feel resistance to this. Why? Because all you know is the current playbook. You may not even be winning at the game of life right now but at least you know the rules so it feels comfortable to you, familiar, secure. You may hate parts of your life right now, like your weight and lack of energy or low self-confidence, but the minute you say you're going to try to change it, the rules kick into high gear.

Have you ever seen a bunch of five-year-olds play a made-up imaginary game where they're creating the rules along the way, and then after fifteen minutes or so one kid wants to change the rules?

"No. That's not how you play the game," says one kid.

"Unfair, you don't get to change the rules," chimes in another.

"Yeah, you can't do that," says a third.

Oh, my goodness. Anarchy.

The original child who wanted to change the rules has one

of two options. She says, "Too bad, this is how we're playing. It'll be more fun," and hopes the other kids will adapt and play with her or, she gives up and says, "Okay, let's just keep playing the way we were."

This is happening in your life all the time. You want to change the rules but the forces of comfort in your life won't let you.

Here's the psychology bit you need to know:

Overwhelm

The minute you think a *new* thought or want to change the rules, you're challenging yourself and the way you're playing the game of life. At this point, your subconscious mind, which doesn't like change at all, is going to generate all sorts of thoughts in your head that cause you to feel fear, doubt, and worry. Fear, doubt, and worry become the predominant emotions that you experience around this new idea. You'll be fearful of failing again, you'll doubt your abilities, and you'll worry about whether or not it's even worth trying to lose weight again when you've tried so many times in the past and failed.

This fear, doubt, and worry can lead to feeling anxious and scattered. You may even feel overwhelmed by this new idea. Overwhelm is a mental construct. It's a decision that you end up making, possibly subconsciously, and it's the precursor to quitting. Feeling overwhelmed is the precursor to quitting. Highlight that phrase so you remember this. The minute you go into overwhelm and don't even realize that you have done this, you've already pretty much lost the change battle and the ability to go on a true weight-loss journey. Your subconscious wins again.

Boo.

Rationalize

At this point you start to rationalize where you are and come up with all sorts of justifiable reasons (ahem… excuses) about why this can't be done right now. And the smarter, more accomplished, driven, and successful you are, the better and more believable your justifiable rationalizations will be because you've been living with these rules longer. Essentially, you've gotten good at lying to yourself.

You'll tell yourself things like:

- This is too hard
- I don't have enough time for this
- I'm too tired
- I'll start this next week… next month… next year
- I'm too busy
- This isn't important right now
- This doesn't matter
- I don't care

Ouch. None of those things are true, but that's your way out. To give yourself enough excuses to not even try so you don't have to fail again.

Blame

Then, if you're like most of my clients, and how I was at one point in my life too, you'll start to play the blame game. You'll blame everything external to yourself about why you can't be successful in this area of your life; health and weight loss.

You'll blame it on your kids' busy schedules, or that you travel a lot for work, or that you're always eating out with clients. You'll blame your life, your genetics, your mom, the fact that you're big boned, or the stage of life that you're in (perimenopause or menopause). You'll blame your hormones, the fact that you have a bad or slow metabolism, or that you can't find enough time to exercise.

Or, you might personalize this and blame yourself for not having enough willpower and discipline but then you justify why you don't, based on the previous list we came up with. It's a vicious cycle.

Old Programming

This takes you right back down the rabbit hole to old programming, living your life on default. Engaging in all of your habits. You go right back to the rules of the game that you've been playing by because it feels safe, familiar, and comfortable to you. Let me be clear: you don't like it but you're willing to endure it. Women are capable of enduring a significant amount of suffering before they become truly willing to change.

You are extremely capable of tolerating your own lies. I mean, you've listened to them for years and you believe them. Heck, you may even convince other people in your life that you're right about yourself, so they now support your story too. This is why weight loss on your own is challenging. It's you versus you. Often, the old you who likes the old rules wins.

When you go on a weight-loss journey what you're saying to yourself is that you want to go to a new destination in your life. It's that you know the rules that you've created in your life have worked up until now but you're craving something new in your life. It means you've got to change the rules because what you have done in the past and the way that you've lived your life up until this point is not going to get you to where you want to go. If it could have, you'd already be there by now and you wouldn't be reading this book.

When you are in the game of transformation, it's a big deal. Weight loss is the most significant, transformative vehicle for a woman because it's deeply personal. It requires you to get back in touch with yourself. To dig up the roots of the dandelions that exist in your subconscious. You need to observe and expose your belief systems and challenge your limiting thoughts, and that is work. Powerful work, necessary work but hard work, nonetheless. Most women will spend decades of their lives trying to lose weight on a diet. They will repeatedly fail until they're willing to go deep. For an outer transformation to happen, you have to do your inner work.

When you become willing to play a different game and change the rules that you've been living your life by, life gets more fun. You start to invite more possibilities and more good opportunities in your life. And that on its own can be scary.

We're into the deep stuff now, aren't we?

There are a lot of other reasons why you know better but don't do better. Many of them are things that you can change but it does mean changing the rules of the game, so you need to become willing.

This is perhaps the most crazy-making thing about weight loss. You know what to do, you just don't do it. Why is that?

Weight loss can easily happen when you take care of the other basic lifestyle factors that influence your overall health, energy level, and feelings of vitality.

Could Lack of Sleep Be Making You Fat?

Yes.

Large scale studies show that consistently not sleeping enough makes you way more likely to put on weight over time. When you sleep less you tend to consume more calories in the form of candy, pop, and junk food throughout the day, and especially at night when you feel tired and want something to help you feel better.

The challenge with getting enough sleep is that so many women tell me that they love that quiet time at night once the kids have gone to bed and the day is done. They feel like it's their time to relax. Most of my clients say things like, "That's *me* time. That's the time of day that I look forward to when I get to sit and chill and have a treat. I deserve that after a long, hard day."

Do you? Because here's what typically happens.

You're exhausted, feel tired, drained, and worn out and you tell yourself you're going to have one square of chocolate. You get it and go sit down on the couch with whatever your favorite show is on Netflix. Before you know it, you've got the chocolate bar wrapper beside you and you've eaten the whole thing, you're now watching the third show even though you intended to only watch one. You finally haul your tired butt to the bedroom to go to bed, but now your mind is focused on what a failure you are and you're lying there feeling your fat, dreading the fact that you have to get up in the morning and start your diet over again.

What gives?

Sleep affects the brain functions that are related to food choices and desire. Researchers have found that when sleep-deprived, the brain responds with a much greater desire for unhealthy food than when rested. As well, a sleep-deprived brain has a diminished capacity to make reasoned, thoughtful decisions because the frontal lobe is no longer functioning optimally. The frontal lobe of your brain is responsible for alertness, attention, decision making, and cognitive processes. Simply put, it becomes difficult to overcome the impulse to eat poorly.

Researchers have discovered by using MRI technology that a sleep-deprived brain when compared to a rested brain will always perform in a more negative way when it comes to food. For instance:

- Even minor sleep deprivation can create a greater desire for unhealthy, empty-calorie foods *and* people will rate their desire for these foods much higher compared to when they're rested.
- The more sleep-deprived people believe they are, the more they wanted junk food.
- The "reward center" of a sleep-deprived brain lights up more when shown pictures of high-calorie foods (junk).
- A sleep-deprived brain has decreased activity in the frontal lobe – the part of the brain that controls complex decision-making and behavior control. That means when sleep-deprived, you'll have much less ability to make good/ healthy decisions for yourself regarding food.

Think about all of this. You're tired and essentially trying to exert willpower or discipline on your diet by not eating something that you're not supposed to have, except to your poor functioning brain that food looks even more enticing and desirable and you have less ability to make a good decision for yourself.

Yikes.

Then, you start the day all over again by hitting snooze in the morning because you're tired and well… it feels like Groundhog Day.

Not sleeping well also affects your ability to handle stress. Stress is another major lifestyle factor that influences whether or not weight loss will happen for you.

Stress

You know that stress isn't good for you, but most women cite feeling stressed out at frequent points throughout the day. There are two types of stress – acute and chronic. Both types of stress can make you reach for comfort foods and sugary treats that stress your body out even more.

Acute stress: this is short-term stress. It's the stress you experience when you're responding to both past and present demands or anticipated demands (i.e., stuck in traffic, a tight work deadline, fought with your partner, big presentation). It can feel stimulating and exhausting.

Chronic stress: this is long-term stress. This is the grinding kind of stress that wears people out day after day, year after year. Chronic stress develops when you have repeated exposure to short-term stresses or when you never see a way out of a miserable situation. It's the stress of unrelenting demands and pressures for seemingly interminable periods.

With no hope, you give up searching for solutions and you become acclimated to living with high stress and don't even realize that you're stressed, you're just used to it. Just because something becomes normal for you does not mean that it's healthy.

There are a million psychological and physiological impacts of living with chronic stress. Here are just a few of them:

- Stress-induced hypertension (high blood pressure)
- Increased risk for heart disease and stroke
- Ulcers (digestion)
- Irregular menstrual cycles in females
- Decreased libido
- Decreased function of your immune system so you have an increased likelihood of infectious diseases – you get sick more often
- Anxiety
- Depression

- Neurological disorders – headaches, forgetfulness, inability to focus, feeling scattered
- Moodiness, irritability
- IBS (irritable bowel syndrome)
- Sleep deprivation
- Increased use of alcohol, drugs, and cigarettes

When living with chronic stress, your body starts to feel as if it's living in hormone soup. Some hormones are over-functioning while others are under-functioning. Your hormones become imbalanced. The chemical messengers in your body no longer communicate with each other well and this can lead to a host of physical health problems. Your body was designed to handle short-term or acute stress and has developed a sophisticated stress response aimed at helping you survive.

Stress Response – the Familiar Hormones

When you encounter a perceived threat, your hypothalamus (a tiny region at the base of your brain) sets off a cascade of events. Through neural and hormonal signals, it prompts your adrenal glands that sit on top of your kidneys to flood your body with hormones – primarily adrenaline and cortisol so that you can be ready to fight-or-flight.

Adrenaline and Norepinephrine:

- Primes you for fight or flight
- Increases your heart rate
- Elevates your blood pressure
- Cortisol:
- Primary stress hormone
- Increases sugar in the bloodstream
- Increases your brain's use of glucose

Stress Response and Glucocorticoids

Glucocorticoids are a group of hormones (cortisol is part of this group) that are released when you're stressed. They remain in your bloodstream for a significant amount of time – even after the stressor is gone. One of their functions is to make sure you have enough energy to handle the stressor and will replenish energy stores by increasing your sugar cravings. They desensitize you to leptin, allowing you to overeat and increase fat storage. Today, you can experience incredible amounts of stress while sitting at a desk, have no energy expenditure happen, yet still experience strong cravings for sugar and fat.

How Does Stress Create Sugar Cravings?

Your stress response directly affects your food intake. Your survival once depended on your body making sure that when you encountered any life-threatening event that you'd have enough energy to survive it. Nowadays, your "stressors" aren't necessarily physically demanding (i.e., worrying about money) but your body doesn't know the difference. When stressed, you may:

- Sleep poorly
- Crave sugar – candy, pop
- Crave carbs – bread, doughy things
- Eat poorly
- Skip meals
- Eat takeout
- Eat late at night
- Eat "treat" foods
- Drink more coffee
- Consume more booze
- Exercise less or exercise more

- Feel like you have less willpower or commitment to your goals so you give up for a few days (or months)
- Stop doing the things you know are good for you

Stress causes you to move into "fight," "flight," "freeze," and "eat" responses. Managing your stress is a critical component to cutting back on sugar cravings and leading a healthy, fit, fulfilling life – rarely is anyone ever taught how to do this.

To lose weight and keep it off, you have to start to recognize your emotional cues and triggers. That's why we have a whole chapter on habits. If you're engaged in self-sabotage because it's your habit or if you sabotage your health with other important lifestyle factors like living sleep-deprived or constantly under a state of stress then weight loss becomes even more difficult. Often a whole life reset is required and diets don't explain that, which is why I had to write this book. Weight loss requires a sane approach which means also understanding why you use food to stuff down feelings you don't feel like feeling.

11

Why Do I Eat My Feelings?

"It's time to inhale courage and exhale fear."
—Jennifer Powter

The biggest fear my clients have is that if they start to feel their feelings, then they'd never stop crying or feeling angry. What if they get lost in their feelings and can never find their way out? So many women live life feeling disconnected – maybe you feel this way, too. Feeling your feelings may have become so painful it was easier to disconnect from them, and that became your habit.

What I like to say is that feelings are like waves in the ocean crashing against the beach. Some waves are big; some waves are small. Some come in big sets which feel unrelenting, then sometimes there's a sea of calm. Feelings are supposed to come and go, but when you don't allow yourself to feel your feelings or if you get stuck in a feeling and begin to form your identity around it, that's when the trouble begins.

Learning how to become fluent in feeling and expressing your emotions is vital to putting an end to emotional eating. And it takes courage. For years, maybe even decades, food has given you a way to numb yourself to your feelings.

You may not like this process, but you need to be committed to it.

Typically, at an early age in life, you were told what was acceptable and what wasn't in terms of your emotions. You also witnessed your parents handle their emotions (or stuff them down) and that set the stage for your adult life.

When you feel emotions that cause pain (grief, anger, disappointment, resentment), it's easy to let food become the drug that helps you stuff them down, but emotional eating creates a different kind of pain in your life and you get trapped in a vicious cycle of trying to escape pain and creating more pain for yourself.

The only way to escape the trap is to have the courage to feel and to establish better coping mechanisms, and it's a process.

- Every thought you think impacts your reality.
- Your known thoughts and feelings perpetuate the same state of being, which creates the same behaviors, and the same reality.
- Why would you think thoughts you don't want to happen in life? Answer: it's your habit.
- Your emotions (or lack of feeling them) have become memorized for you and have created your personality. Now you're changing that.
- It's easy to focus on behaviors, but now it's time to go deeper into aligning your thoughts and feelings in what you want most.
- You can't create change when you hang on to skepticism, cynicism, self-doubt, worry, fear, self-loathing, anger, and resentment.

You are here on this planet to live fully and love deeply. Emotional eating has been your way of trying to take care of yourself. By now, you're seeing that the way you use food has been to stuff down the feelings you haven't known what to do with.

You've done the work to learn what it is you're feeling and may have a strong intellectual understanding of the emotions you're experiencing, but now you need to learn the art of reflecting on these emotions and developing a healthy way to express your emotions, not just talk about them.

The Truth About Your Feelings

Ever since you were little you were taught to be distracted from your feelings. To see this in real life just go to a shopping mall and watch how parents handle their children when their child is upset, mad, or frustrated. The child starts to express an emotion and immediately the distraction techniques come out. For babies a soother or bottle gets stuffed in its mouth or a rattle or phone gets pulled out. For toddlers, there's the promise of ice cream or candy "if they're good."

For older kids the expression of their feelings may be met with contempt or judgment: "Are you seriously going to start complaining? You should be grateful for what you've got," or "Honestly, I don't want to hear one more word from you. Just shut up." Look for the pain and confusion on that child's face. They were simply trying to express an emotion. In our culture we've labeled emotions as positive or negative but here's the truth about your feelings:

- All feelings are essential whether they feel good or distressing to experience
- Feelings give you important information about your life and how it's working for you
- Feelings are the primary motivating force in your life

- Without acknowledging your core feelings, you lose your sense of "self," start to feel like a "shell of who you once were," or "numb"

You eat because your survival depends on it, but that's not the only reason. Over time, eating has become a way of coping – a way to anesthetize yourself to the pain in life. Food can become a band-aid and give you something you think you need, want or desire, but the ache always returns.

Emotional eating is common. But it is just a symptom of a deeper problem. When you learn what it is you need and want *most* in life *and* take the action to create that for yourself, it's amazing how much your attachment to food or booze lessens.

There are some basic reasons that you eat beyond just fueling your body with energy. Read these and see which ones resonate as true for you.

You Eat for Pleasure/Fun/Entertainment

Quite frankly, you might be bored with your life and eating gives you something to do. Perhaps this is because you're in a job that you hate and you have to do things that you find boring so you take a break and go distract yourself with food. It provides some relief from the boredom, but that relief is temporary. Maybe you go home to an empty house and you sit and watch TV. You don't have any hobbies or activities that you're involved with and so you're bored at night. You sit and eat. Or perhaps you're bored in your relationship. There's no spark, no connection, no physical or emotional intimacy, so perhaps you and your partner pretend that you're not bored by eating together. It provides you both with a few moments of joy but that's all. Eventually, you go back to feeling bored in your relationship.

Many of my clients are bored. Somehow, with the grind of adulthood, their life has gotten small, they've stopped doing things that they love, opted out of extracurricular activities and feel a sense of blah-ness during their days or evenings. There's simply not much going on or to look forward to, so eating provides some pleasure.

You Eat to Give You a Break in Your Day or to Provide Yourself with a Transition Activity

Mary is a school teacher. She loved her evening gin and a tonic cocktail at 5:30 p.m. because it meant her day was done and that she could now relax. To her, the alcoholic cocktail meant she could put her work away for the day and have some fun. It's easy to let food or booze become associated as a transition activity; it's a justifiable reason to move from one part of your day to another.

Shania typically got to work at 7 a.m. She works in a big energy company downtown and likes to beat the traffic and get an early start on her work. Around 10 a.m., she'd pop over to her colleagues' cubicle pod and the three or four of them would take a break together and go to Starbucks where she'd order a latte and a baked good (usually the cinnamon coffee cake). That was her break in the morning and she looked forward to it. It was a one-block walk and the group would talk and laugh as they spent time together.

For Maggie, it was enjoying a bowl of cereal before bed. That's what her mom always used to give her and her sister when they were little and it became her habit. She told me it made her feel cozy and safe and that when her cereal was done it was time for bed.

All of the above examples are about using food or drinks as a transition activity so that you know it's time to move from one part of your day to the next. The problem is that this provides your body with a boatload of unnecessary calories and contributes to your weight loss problem. When you think about dieting or trying to lose weight, often these kinds of habits are the ones that are hardest to change because you enjoy the feelings you get from doing them.

You Eat to Feel a Sense of Security

This is a common habit if you came from a home that had lots of instability in it when you were younger. Often, food became a thing that helped distract you from your anxiety or fear. As a child, mom and dad might be fighting but you snuck the bag of marshmallows into your room to share with you and your little brother to distract you guys from what was going on in your home. This kind of early association with food can have a hangover effect in your adult years.

Perhaps now, when you find yourself in uncomfortable situations you make yourself busy in the kitchen cooking and/or eating. Eating makes you busy. It gives you an excuse to hide, not engage, not talk, and not participate.

Food and alcohol can also become a source of emotional stamina. It's like a bandage when in a stressful situation. I can't tell you the number of times I've heard, "I just need a glass of wine to help get me through this." Or there are the scenes in the movies where the character needs a good dose of courage so she downs two shots and off she goes to do whatever it is. And we've all seen the sign, "Yes, you can dance. Vodka tells you so."

You Eat Because Food Gives You Protection

I don't believe my clients see this in themselves at first, but after it's pointed out or discussed they all say, "Yes. I do that." Food becomes such a justifiable way to avoid things in your life. It's like the perfect avoidance strategy. Anytime you're faced with a situation you don't like or are experiencing emotions that don't feel good, you've got an out for dealing with them by deciding that you're hungry and need to eat.

It was way easier for me to pour a glass of wine and eat some chocolate, believing that I deserved a treat than it was for me to face the fact that my marriage was in a breakdown. I was lonely and scared of getting divorced and becoming a single parent. Who wants to face that? I've heard similar stories from women who were taking care of a sick parent or child or who were sick themselves. Instead of dealing with painful emotions, they felt they were able to distract themselves with food (or wine). But ultimately, you can't hide from the truth of what's going on for you in your life. You may try, but I say this is akin to an ostrich sticking its head in the sand during a sandstorm. While it may have its head in the sandstorm and pretend that everything is fine, the storm is still raging on around her. Eventually, she'll need to look up.

This doesn't have to be just emotional avoidance. Eating can be a great way to avoid unpleasant tasks that you are simply required to do in your work or life. I remember when I first started working from home and needed to write my email newsletter. I didn't believe I was a good writer and I hated doing the task. Coincidentally enough, I always found myself hungry when I was supposed to write. I'd go make a snack, eat it, and then go back to my desk. I'd still feel hungry, so I'd go make something else. It didn't change the fact that my writing task was still there for me. What I discovered is that this happens to lots of women. The more undesirable something is to you, the more you'll try to avoid doing it. Being hungry and needing to eat is the perfect excuse to not do something you don't feel like doing.

There are deeper emotional reasons that you eat when you're not truly hungry. Here are the more common ones:

Eating Helps You Feel Connection

As you become an adult, often the range of activities that you're involved in and your free time decrease dramatically due to family and work demands. Going out for dinner, lunch, or Sunday brunch, or texting a girlfriend to grab a drink with you after work is the perfect activity to do – after all, you need to eat. Food becomes a way to connect with people in your life. It can give you an excuse or reason to call someone and see if they want to get together. In some ways, it's a way to protect yourself. If they reject you, they can make it that lunch/dinner doesn't work for them, not that they don't want to see you.

It's a way to feel close to someone, to do what they're doing. To feel validated and like you're a part of something. This happens a lot on the weekends with women and can be one of the (sub)conscious fears that exist around losing weight. There's a fear that you'll lose your social life.

Thursday nights were the highlight of Colleen's week. She told me that she and five or six girlfriends would meet at their favorite bar for a drink and then stay and have dinner together. Her husband knew that this was "her night out" and that he was on "home-duty" with the kids. She described this night as an epic, free-for-all where it wasn't uncommon to have six to eight drinks, greasy, cheesy, fried appetizers, a full dinner, and then share a dessert. This was her cheat night, and she was terrified I was going to take it away from her when we started working together. At first, she didn't mention the horrible two-day hangover that made her snarky and irritable with her family or how she would go all day Friday without eating to make up for everything she ate the night before. She just talked about how much fun she had with her girlfriends.

Can you spot the challenge here? Colleen had blended food and booze and having fun into one collective experience. It was as if she gave up one thing, the entire night would be different. She feared that her girlfriends wouldn't find her as much fun, she wouldn't be able to truly relax and enjoy herself, and she wouldn't get the "break" that she needed from her exhausting home life.

Her girlfriends were also overweight. She said that she didn't want to make them feel bad about themselves by changing her behavior and losing weight. She believed it was just easier to go along and do what they were doing because she didn't want to stand out or draw attention to herself or her weight loss goal. This one night out a week undid everything else Colleen was doing. But she didn't know that.

Colleen finally decided that enough was enough. She no longer wanted to feel this way or live her life like this. She made a commitment to herself and has never looked back. She spoke honestly to her girlfriends about how she felt and shared vulnerably that she needed their support. She asked if they could change up what they did on Thursday nights so engaging in self-sabotaging behaviors wouldn't be so tempting. They all agreed. In fact, every woman in that circle of friends told Colleen that they admired her and wanted to be healthier too. Colleen has lost twenty-eight pounds and can now shop her own closet because everything fits again.

You Want to Keep the Peace, so You Engage in People-Pleasing Behavior

Have you ever said yes to something when you wanted to say no? What about eating something you didn't enjoy simply because someone else made it for you or gave you some? If you answered

145

yes to either of these questions, chances are you engage in people-pleasing behaviors as a way to avoid conflict. It simply seems easier for you to do this and avoid the potential of upsetting someone else. It's like you operate with the idea that keeping the peace is the most important thing, and you become willing to sacrifice yourself or goals to do it. While it may be an effective strategy in the short-term, it kicks you in the butt down the road. Why? Because most of the time you're making up a story about what you think people need and want from you and for you and you're going to be wrong most of the time.

It can look like going home for the holidays and eating the pumpkin pie because mom made it especially for you because it's your favorite (you don't even like pumpkin pie and never did as a kid). At first, you say no thank you, but then you see the slight hurt, concerned look cross your mom's face as she asks you if you're okay. You say you're fine. She then goes on to say that she spent the whole day making the pie for you and asks again if you're sure you don't want any. At this point, you're feeling uncomfortable with the situation, and because you love your mom and have a huge heart, you say, "You know what, mom? I'd love a slice." And you choke it down along with some bitterness and resentment that you're once again trying to please someone else. After you eat the pie, you think "to heck with it" and go get some ice cream too. You've already blown your diet, might as well make it worth it.

The Blame Game Justifies Your Eating Behavior

This is about to whack you upside the head because this happens for most of my clients. They eat way more than they need to and then blame other people or situations for why they did what they did. If I've heard one of these a million times I've heard all of them. When you blame situations outside of yourself, you grant yourself permission to sneakily justify and rationalize your behavior. The most common phrase I hear is:

"Well it's not my fault, I mean…"

- I was on vacation
- It was my birthday
- It was the holidays
- I was sick
- I was so stressed due to work
- I was traveling for work

Any time you say, "I couldn't help it," what you're saying is, "I didn't want to help it."

And take a good look at those "reasons." I promise you that if you don't choose to get in the driver seat of your life and take control of your health, choices, boundaries and see all of that as a radical act of self-love then your weight issues will plague you forever.

Last time I checked, you're probably always going to go on a few vacations a year and if you're like me your monthly calendar is filled with friends' and family members' birthdays. There's pretty much a holiday or special event day every month (Christmas, Hanukkah, winter break, Valentine's Day, spring break, Easter, St. Patrick's Day, Memorial Day weekend, end-of-year school parties, summer holidays/potlucks/BBQs, camping season, Labor Day weekend, Halloween, Thanksgiving, and we're right back to Christmas).

If you're living life by burning the candle at both ends and not getting good quality sleep and feeling stressed out, we've already talked about how that impairs your immune system so getting sick is more likely (when you're sick you crave comfort foods) and ta-da – there's your excuse.

Honestly, I just had a friend text me asking if I could come over for a glass of wine (it's currently 3 p.m.). Her text then said, "I mean, it's Thursday and it's wine o'clock somewhere!" Excuses to justify what you do are all around you.

You Eat to Escape and to Avoid Feeling

Most women eat to numb out and avoid their feelings. I had one client, Anna, tell me the more she stuffed in her mouth, the further she stuffed her feelings down. The bigger the feelings, the more she ate. At the time, she was going through a divorce. Her husband left her. To not feel that rejection, she ate and ate and ate.

You may have learned this behavior when you were young. If you had a family that didn't like "unpleasant emotions" (I don't think there's any such thing. But some families don't leave a lot of room for anger or sadness, they just want everyone to be happy), then perhaps every time you were sad, your mom took you to the kitchen and suggested making cookies to cheer you up. Or maybe you fell and skinned your knee and you were given ice cream to take the pain away. What seems so innocent can create a lifetime of complications with food.

As a baby, one of the ways you got nurtured was by being held and fed. As an adult, it's time to learn other, more effective ways to nurture yourself as food is meant to nourish you, not be an emotional crutch or escape tool.

Learning to Nurture Yourself

You know when you have a crap day and things just feel hard? You wish you had someone to hug you, make you some soup, and just take care of you – that is the desire to be nurtured.

It makes sense that when you look for a way to ease the emotional burdens, you turn to food; it's quick, always available, and can fill the gap (bandage).

Create Your Own Emotional Safety

- A sense of emotional safety is the base of your nurturing as it makes you feel protected, strong, and secure
- You get to develop this for yourself but to do so you need to slow down and focus on creating rituals and routines for yourself that don't include food
- When you create and follow healthy routines and rituals, you're nurturing yourself

Women don't have weight problems. They have self-esteem and self-loathing problems. They have habits of self-neglect and self-abandonment. They have integrity and accountability challenges. They have unhealed trauma from the past that they need to deal with. I don't just mean big T trauma like sexual or physical abuse. They have issues with creating and maintaining boundaries. They're suffering from an inability to handle the busy-ness of their lives and they keep adding more on instead of taking things away. Typically, all of the above gets bundled under a weight problem. Why? Because these are the real reasons you overeat and that's the real reason you're overweight.

At some point, life got the better of you. By the time you hit your forties, chances are you went through some hard things. Divorce, betrayal, heartbreak, financial crisis, taking care of kids, nursing a sick parent, or suffered a devastating loss.

Maybe it was the loss of your dreams, your ambition, or the vision that you had for your life, and now you're wondering, "Is this it?" You're a good person who is kind and generous and yet somehow you get the short end of the stick. Life doesn't feel fair. And your weight is like salt on a wound. The beauty is that you always have the power of choice and your past does not predict your future. Every moment gets to be a new moment and you get to decide what you want to create for yourself, your health, your weight and your life.

This is the weight loss "inner work" that most women want to skip over. Why? Because it takes energy and requires you to ask yourself some tough questions and answer them. I want to make this simple for you. It's time to take stock of what's going on for you. Do not skip over this part. Pull out your journal and get ready to write. It's time to dissect your behavior and to take care of the things that you've been tolerating in your life that are not serving you and are keeping you trapped in a relationship with food and your weight that you hate. Trust me, what you are tolerating is one of the key reasons you are eating your feelings. It's time for that to stop.

What Are You Tolerating?

The easiest way to move into action is to identify what you've been tolerating in your life and deal with some of those things. It's amazing how we trick ourselves into believing that "that's just the way things are" or "I'll do that later" or "That doesn't matter" when often that's not the truth at all. You've simply forgotten how capable you are.

The definition of "tolerate" is:

- Allow the existence, occurrence, or practice of (something that one does not necessarily like or agree with) without interference
- Accept or endure (someone or something unpleasant or disliked) with forbearance
- Be capable of continued subjection to (a drug, toxin or environmental condition) without adverse reaction

I can guarantee there are things in your life that you tolerate. Somehow that mean voice inside your head has seduced you into believing that it's better to avoid something than deal with it, that you should just "suck it up," or maybe even has you fearful about something so you procrastinate and avoid instead.

These could be:

- You're tolerating a messy car
- You're tolerating old towels in your bathroom when you'd like new ones
- You're tolerating hating your clothes
- You're tolerating not paying your bills on time
- You're tolerating relationships that are unhappy and unfulfilling
- You're tolerating being lonely
- You're tolerating feeling so busy
- You're tolerating a messy fridge
- You're tolerating keeping quiet
- You're tolerating your job

Everything that you tolerate creates stress in your life. That chronic, low-grade kind of stress that isn't enough to motivate you to do something about it but is having an effect on you both emotionally and physically. Often this kind of stress is what drives you to eat in order to get some relief or comfort or the ability to escape. Over and over I have found that when my clients start to take action on the things they've tolerated, their weight-loss journey gets easier and easier.

This was certainly true for Brenda. Brenda was a corporate attorney who had two teenage boys who played hockey. She was (mostly) happily married but was running around ragged and her weight had spiraled out of control in the past decade. She came to me at her all-time heaviest of 227 pounds. "I have no idea where to start or what to do but I know that I can't continue to exist this way. All of my clothes are tight, and I refuse to size-up again. Everybody seems to need me, and I can't give enough. I'm tired."

When it came time to identifying what Brenda tolerated, she was resistant. She said things like, "Well, that's just how it is," and I had to keep reminding her that no, that's just how she allowed it to be. She started to write and by the time she had dumped her brain onto paper she had 104 things that she identified she was "tolerating" in her life.

Things like organizing her kids' hockey gear, doing all of the laundry, people not respecting her time and being late to meetings, working weekends, old makeup, on and on the list went. She couldn't believe how much energy she used up pretending that these things didn't matter. Brenda could hear the times she told herself that she deserved a glass of wine or a cookie for dealing with what she was choosing to tolerate.

The last time we spoke, Brenda had eighteen things left on her list of tolerations, she's lost thirty-one pounds (she hasn't been under 200 pounds for fifteen years), and has radically decreased the stress she was experiencing in her life. She took action. It started small and the wins got bigger and bigger.

Now it's your turn.

Write down everything that you're currently tolerating, and I mean everything. It could be things about yourself, your environment, or your relationships. It could be big things like you're tolerating a job that you hate and a relationship that you're unfulfilled in, to little things like the chaos in your laundry room, or mismatched socks in your sock drawer. Pick two things and do something about it. Then pick another two, and another two.

You already know that taking action creates mini-wins, this increases your confidence which helps you take more action and helps you build momentum. Things that were hard get easier.

Now that you've identified what you've been tolerating, it's time to get clear on what you love and enjoy. Sometimes this is harder than figuring out what you've been tolerating. The goal here is to remind yourself of all of the non-food ways you can create amazing experiences for yourself in your life and begin to nurture yourself in kind, loving ways. Here are some questions to get you going:

- What was your favorite activity as a kid?
- When do you laugh the most? What are you doing?
- What could you spend hours doing?
- When have you felt most alive in your life? What were you up to?
- What's your current favorite hobby? (Hint: if you don't have one that's ok, what have you always wanted to try doing?)
- What brings you joy? (Sunshine? Flowers? Warm cup of tea?)
- When/where do you feel most relaxed?
- What's your favorite way to have fun?
- What have you always wanted to do but have been too busy?

These questions are meant to be a springboard for your brain to help remind yourself of activities that you could do that would bring a sense of emotional relief, fulfillment or reward into your life. When you start to create a life that feels fulfilling to you, a life that you enjoy and have fun in, it's amazing how the desire to numb disappears because you no longer are "coping" with your life, you're living it and enjoying it.

Once you understand the real reasons you turn to food, to avoid feeling your feelings, it's easier to create change in your life because you're now getting to the root of your weight loss issues. That said, most people have little understanding of food, nutrition or the impact that liquid calories have on your body.

Honestly, it was shocking for me to realize that a four-ounce glass of wine was about the same calorie count as a piece of bread. Sure, it was metabolized differently but that meant there were some nights when I drank two eight-ounce glasses of wine I was consuming the equivalent of four and a half pieces of bread (calorie-wise)! No wonder I couldn't lose weight! The next chapter explains the general concepts of macronutrients and why it's important to choose your food, not cheat with it.

12

Back to the Basics with Food

"I stopped waiting for the light at the end
of the tunnel and lit my own torch."
—Unknown

We live in a world of instant gratification. Everything is at the click of a button or flip of a switch, and I know you want weight loss to be the same. You want it to be fast so that you can feel good about yourself again. That's exactly how the weight loss industry grew to be a $70 billion industry. It's full of fourteen-day cleanses, fad diets, and supplement-driven products that all say you can lose weight quickly. Sometimes you do. But quick and dirty weight loss leads to quick and dirty weight regain. Fast, healthy, permanent weight loss doesn't exist.

There are some basic elements of weight loss that got lost in the noise of the dieting industry. Misinformation gets spread around like a virus and at the end of the day, you feel like you don't even know what's true and what's not.

There are two critical things to understand when it comes to permanent weight loss. The first is understanding food and how it impacts your body. The second is understanding the psychology of behavior change which we've already talked about a fair bit. This is going to be the science-y section. But you need to know this or else it's like expecting to be able to go to France and have conversations with the French people, but it's frustrating because you don't know the language and you aren't fluent yet.

Most women don't understand the simple elements of food and sometimes they even become afraid of certain food groups (that's right, carbs). Maybe you've been told that to lose weight you have to go keto, paleo or give up all carbs forever. And you've tried. You've experienced the headaches, the cravings and eventually crumbled under the desire to simply eat a food that you want.

Let's make it simple.

First, you have to understand what is driving your body's engine. That's called your basal metabolic rate. This term refers to the number of calories required to keep your body functioning at rest. Four factors influence how much energy you need: height, weight, gender and the amount of muscle mass you have on your body.

Remember the "kitty cat versus lion" metaphor? The bigger you are, the more calories you need to sustain life. This is why no cookie-cutter diet formula works for all women.

A woman who is 5'8" tall, is over 230 pounds, and used to be an athlete so has a high amount of muscle mass on her body needs to eat more food than a woman who is 5'1", 170 pounds, and has little muscle mass on her body.

It's not because she has a bad metabolism. It's not because her body is broken or she has bad genetics.

It's not because of her hormones.

It's because she is petite.

Nothing makes me more frustrated than women trying to lose weight and blaming their perfectly amazing bodies and getting down on themselves. If you just understood what was going on at a physiological level, it would make more sense and you wouldn't get as frustrated and that would allow you to be more successful.

To all of you women out there who are 5'4" or less – let me tell you something. Weight loss is different for you. That's a fact. It may seem like you gain weight quickly and lose weight slowly, well, that's true. You do. That's what it's like for petite women. For you taller women out there, you have a bit more freedom with weight loss because of your size. You're taller, which influences your basal metabolic rate, meaning you require more energy (calories) to function.

When you're a mini-kitty (5'4" and under), you have to remember that you live in a lion-sized world. It may feel restrictive that you don't get to eat the same way as your husband or friends but it's due to your physiology that this true. Not because your body is broken.

I teach live workshops to women and at one of my events in Calgary, there was a woman named Joanie who was 4'11." I taught my kitty cat versus lion metaphor, and all of a sudden, everything clicked for her. She jumped and said excitedly, "I'm not failing. I just didn't know so I've been overeating. This is freedom to realize my body isn't broken; I just didn't know what it needed." She then went on to lose thirty pounds by changing how much she ate in a day. She ate like a mini-kitty instead of a lion.

So often women beat themselves up for a lack of weight loss success when they simply don't know the basics of how to lose weight. We've already gone through why exercise isn't the answer as you can't out-train your fork, but now it's time to explain why understanding food, and how much to eat, is critical to losing weight.

Know Your Macros

There are three basic macronutrients, which are the nutrients you need in large amounts, as they provide your body with the calories it needs to function properly. The basic macronutrients are carbohydrates, protein, and fat.

Carbohydrates provide energy and fuel the body just like gasoline fuels a car. Carbs help us function and give us the energy to do things. Carbs include things like pasta, bread, rice, potatoes, oats, cereals, and fruit.

Proteins provide the body with amino acids, which are the essential building blocks that are needed for growth, development, and repair of the body. We need protein to help repair muscle, keep our immune system healthy, and fight inflammation and infection. Typical proteins are things like meat/fish/poultry items, or Greek yogurt, cottage cheese, tofu, and eggs.

Fats are another essential macronutrient. Fats support cell growth, protect your organs, contribute to hormone production, and help your body to absorb some nutrients. Fats include things like all oils, cheese, and nuts.

There is another classification called micronutrients which include vitamins and minerals. They are essential for good health but they don't provide any calories and only trace amounts are needed. Getting enough of the proper vitamins and minerals is critical for your body to function properly.

All three macronutrients are essential but most women are fearful of carbs. They blame carbs on either their weight gain or inability to lose weight. This is how carb-free or low-carb diets became so popular. But carbs aren't necessarily to blame. It's *not* understanding all of the three macronutrients and how they work to support good health and weight loss that's the issue.

Most women who come to me for weight loss are protein deficient, fiber deficient, overeat fats and eat way more carbs than they should for the size that they are, you know, kitty cat size. Once we balance out the macronutrients and determine how much is enough for their kitty cat body, things get a whole lot simpler, and weight loss becomes easier.

You see, carbs can fall under two categories – the "simple carbs" and the "complex carbs." The complex carbs are things like sweet potatoes, brown rice, quinoa, and whole wheat bread which provide long-term energy for the body. Complex carbs contain the fiber found naturally in the food (that's a good thing). The simple carbohydrates or refined carbohydrates (think processed food) include things like white rice, white pasta, white bread, candy, granola bars, cookies, pop, and juice. The fiber has been stripped out of these refined carbs and it's these types of carbohydrates that negatively affect weight gain or inability to lose weight.

Why? Because simple carbohydrates cause major hormone fluctuations in the body as they tend to cause major spikes in blood sugar levels (the sugar high) followed by a sugar crash which can trigger even more sugar/carb cravings. This creates the blood sugar roller coaster for many women.

The body does everything it can to maintain homeostasis, so the minute that blood sugar gets too high, the pancreas is stimulated to release insulin. Insulin is known as the "fat storage" hormone of the body. It tells specific cells in your body to open up and let sugar (glucose) in. Once those cells are full, if there is still *excess* glucose in your bloodstream then that has to be dealt with. The only option now that the glucose storage containers are full is for that sugar to be taken up by your fat cells and stored there for later use.

The problem here is if you continue to overeat, those fat storage containers are never called upon for their energy. Instead, they're asked to store more excess energy. So the fat cells get bigger. What's crazy about fat cells is once they get to their maximum storage quantity and can't hold anymore, new tiny fat cells get created. And now those become the new storage tanks for extra energy that is consumed.

Let's remember a few critical details here – your body is brilliant. Seriously, it's the most incredible vessel on the planet. Like, truly think about it. It allows your heart to pump and you to breathe without thinking about it. It can take two cells and make a baby that stores in your body for nine months. When you get cut, it knows how to heal and repair the tissue. All of that is incredible.

So, when you eat, the body goes to work and starts the process of digestion. All of the nutrients from the foods that you are eating get broken down into little tiny units that the body knows what to do with. When you overeat, the body has *no* choice but to store the leftover calories as fat.

Women talk about fat with a certain tone and distaste. They hate the word and when it's spoken, it usually has a harsh sound to it. Fat. Fat. Fat. But fat is just extra energy that has come onto the body. All of that excess energy is being stored as fat but it's ready to go to work for you at any time. You just have to give it the right signal so that it can become mobilized as a fuel source. The problem is that you don't know how to do that.

Let's look at it this way: you drive your car to the gas station to get gas. You fill up the tank to capacity. And then you also fill up a few jerry cans with gas (fuel for your vehicle) and put them in the back of your car. You are now carrying around extra fuel for your car which you can use at any time. But instead of using those jerry cans which are right there, you keep stopping at the gas station and "topping up." You keep your car's gas tank full at all times which means you never use the jerry cans. This is just like your body.

If you keep eating more than your kitty cat body size needs, overeating, and/or emotional eating, then you never allow fat to be your friend and go to work for you as a fuel source. Instead, you'll hate that fat and punish yourself because you have extra fat on your body and you'll continue to try horrible diets that you put in you a bad headspace because you don't know what else to do.

Here's where women go wrong with carbohydrates. Let's address some simple truths here. Carbs are often quick, crunchy, salty, easy to eat, and become a common grab-and-go snack or the simple thing to eat when you are hungry. If you are trying to get full from eating carbohydrates, you will stay overweight. That is not their job. Their job is to give you the appropriate amount of energy that you need for your size but because they taste so good, you overeat them.

This is where the other macronutrients are so important.

Balancing out your diet with proteins and healthy fats as well as eating a boatload of vegetables is essential for weight loss.

Eat Your Vegetables and Lots of Them

Vegetables contain a boatload of vitamins and minerals – the essential micronutrients that you need for good health *and* weight loss. When I go over my client's food diary and examine what they're eating, they are often vegetable deficient. When I point this out, it's not uncommon to hear, "Well, I don't like vegetables."

I typically say, "What are you, two years old?"

I don't care if you don't like veggies; learn to love them. I tell all of my clients to cultivate a hot, passionate love affair with veggies. Listen, I know that not everyone had a great experience with vegetables as a kid. I can still remember my mom boiling broccoli until it practically turned grey and had this horrendous mush texture to it, but that's in the past.

There are so many ways to prepare vegetables – you can steam, grill, roast, or sauté them. You can have them raw, mix them in a salad, or throw them into the oven. There are so many different ways to season vegetables, it's simply time to experiment. Here's why: if you don't learn to love vegetables, you will never, ever create healthy weight loss for yourself. Vegetables are what allow you to feel full, provide the micronutrients that you need so your body can function properly and prevent a gazillion diseases that are likely to occur if you continue to eat a bad diet.

Did you know that it can take fourteen exposures to one single food for a baby to learn to like it? Create a veggie challenge with yourself and start to increase the quantity that you eat during the week. Experiment with new vegetables. Try to eat the color of the rainbow with vegetables: red, yellow, orange, green, and purple (there aren't many blue veggies). I tend to eat about six to eight cups of vegetables a day. I love them.

Get Your Protein in Throughout the Day

I once read that if you don't get enough protein by 2 p.m. you will consume twice as many carbohydrates at night. Anecdotally, this seems to be true. Many women tend to only eat protein at dinner or in minimal quantities throughout the day. Most Americans eat three times more protein at dinner than breakfast. Scientists recommend spreading protein intake evenly across the day. This means eating roughly twenty-five to thirty grams of protein per meal. Doing so helps to prevent muscle loss with age which is super important as muscle mass influences your basal metabolic rate. Eating protein throughout the day also allows you to feel more full at meals, and prevents sugar cravings or carb cravings which ultimately leads to weight loss.

How to Make Weight Loss Simple

I'm going to make this simple. Eat real food. Stop eating out of a bag, box, or anything that has a wrapper on it. When you limit your processed food and increase the real food that you eat, you will start to nourish yourself. Nourishing yourself physically means that you are better prepared to handle your day. As stress eating diminishes, emotional eating decreases. And that means you aren't overfilling your storage tanks anymore. This is when fat loss can start to happen.

How Much Food Is Enough?

I help every client I work with determine the exact amount of food she needs to nourish herself physically, mobilize fat stores so weight loss can happen, and I do this without putting her on a diet. Women don't need to diet; they need to stop over-eating. The biggest question I get when I present at my live events is, "Well, how much do I need?" That's beyond the scope of this book but here are some simple strategies I can share with you.

1. In Japan, they say, "Hara Hachi Bu," which means stop eating when you're 80 percent full. In our culture, we joke about eating till we're stuffed or putting on our stretchy pants if we're going to a buffet or if it's a big holiday dinner. Start to get connected to your body and determine when you're 80 percent full.

2. Enjoy the foods that you like and simply take less. Remember at all times that you are a kitty cat and just need a kitty cat portion.

3. Forget the word diet. It has the word die in it which I think should tell us something and instead start to practice the LIVE-IT principle which is to eat now with your future lifestyle in mind.

You can't expect to be successful at long-term weight loss if what you're doing right now is hard work. You have to be committed to building a lifestyle for yourself.

I eat whatever I want, whenever I want because I've done my emotional work, food/wine no longer has a grip on me, and I know exactly how much food I need to stay at my ideal weight.

Make Choices. Don't Cheat.

I cannot stand the words "cheat meal" or "cheat day." I hate them. They are horrible principles to live by and 100 percent set you up to fail with weight loss. Stop using them now. I can't tell you how many clients I've had in tears as they explain to me all of the ways they've been trying to lose weight and then they talk about their "cheat meal." I want to lose my mind.

This one cheat meal or cheat day can blow the previous weeks' worth of effort to eat well. Clients have consumed thousands and thousands of calories during a meal like this and this can instantly lead to the scale shooting upward the next day due to water retention, sodium, and excess carb consumption, you can feel bloated, constipated, and worse: you can feel regret.

When you live life on a diet, feeling restricted and deprived, not getting to eat the things that you want but you know that you have a cheat day or meal coming up, then all of your energy goes into thinking about what you're going to have that day. You start to plan, dream and fantasize about all of these forbidden foods and the order that you're going to consume them in. You white-knuckle your way through the week and then let 'er rip on your cheat meal, undoing any weight loss progress you may have been making.

This is weight loss sabotage at its finest. It messes you up both physiologically and psychologically. Even the word "cheat" has horrible meaning – it means to behave in a dishonest way to get what you want. *Say what?* Why would you do this to yourself? Why would you want to create such an awful relationship with food? There is *nothing* healthy about this.

Stop cheating with food and simply *choose* it and accept the consequences of your choices. That's what weight loss is all about. Understanding what you're eating and the impact it will have on your body. On that note, let's talk about choices and consequences.

If you choose:

- To not eat veggies, you're choosing to suffer from carb cravings and slow weight loss
- To eat lion-sized servings, you're choosing to gain weight
- To not spread your protein consumption out throughout the day, you're choosing to make weight loss more difficult for yourself
- If you choose to diet, you're choosing to yo-yo forever
- If you choose to overeat carbohydrates, you're choosing to increase your fat stores
- If you choose to eat take-out, restaurant, or processed foods daily, you're choosing to gain weight

It's time to make better choices. You deserve it. You can do it.

Lastly, learn how to read a food label. If you choose to not learn this critical skill then you are choosing to stay ignorant. You have to know what you're eating. You have to know the amount or proper amount that is a serving. Look at the serving size and number of servings in a bag or a box. Look at how many grams of carbohydrates, fats, and protein are in each serving. Get as knowledgeable about food as you are about money. You know the value of $10, $50 and $100 bills. You understand the concept of a money budget and the consequences of not managing your money appropriately.

It's time to start managing food appropriately and to have intimate knowledge of the quality of the food you're putting in your body and the impact your food choices have on weight loss. The easiest way to do this is to keep a food diary. Your food diary should include the following pieces of information:

- What are you eating? Be specific – write down everything including sauces, toppings, and extras.
- How much: Record the quantity or serving size of the food/drink. This could be measured in volume (one-half cup), weight (three ounces), or the number of items (ten crackers).
- When: Keep track of the time of day.
- Where: Make a note of where you eat. If you're at home is it at the table, in the TV room or at your desk. Write down the names of restaurants you go to.
- Who are you with? Are you alone, or with colleagues, friends or family members?
- Mood Before Eating: How are you feeling when you eat?
- Mood After Eating: What feelings are you experiencing?

Write down every single thing you eat for a week. Do this in real-time otherwise you'll be trying to remember what you ate at the end of the day and you're likely to forget some things.

Write every morsel down – my clients know that in my world "if you bite it, you write it" – it helps you stay honest with yourself.

At the end of the week take a good look at your food diary and spend some time truly looking at how you eat. Things to reflect on are:

- Notice any patterns in your behavior.
- Where can you see easy areas for improvement.
- Are there big gaps between meals?
- Do you tend to skip meals?
- What's your liquid calorie consumption like?
- How much sugar do you typically consume in a day?
- Are you an evening snacker? What do you couple eating with? Watching TV or work?

Food logs or journals can be an effective way to hold yourself accountable and help you create better habits by simply becoming more aware of how, what, when, and why you eat. As you do this, there's a strong likelihood that you'll be able to create a more positive relationship with food and yourself. After all, the relationship you have with yourself is the most important relationship in your life. In the next chapter I explain exactly why discovering the real reasons you're overweight and wanting to release the weight for good can be the gift of a lifetime.

13

Pack Your Bags, You're Going on a Journey

*"Not all storms come to disrupt your
life, some come to clear your path."*
—Unknown

For so many women, weight loss is like death by a thousand cuts. It hurts. I believe that so much of this stems from dieting culture and the relationship that women end up creating with themselves. It's a relationship that is based on lies, distrust, self-betrayal, skepticism, and cynicism. Think about it. How many times have you told yourself that you were going to not eat that thing or drink that drink and then you did? Or all of the times that you said you were going to get up early and work out but then you hit snooze. The times that you said, "Screw it, I don't care," except you do.

The most important relationship you will ever have in your life will be the one that you have with yourself. Most women I know are in horrible relationships with themselves. They say mean things, lie to themselves, say one thing and do another, and over the years this breeds a lack of trust, conviction, and confidence in yourself. No wonder you're not sure if you can lose weight. But let me be clear. You don't have a weight loss problem. You have an integrity problem. You have a problem with follow-through, you have a commitment-to-yourself problem. You have pain and trauma from your past that you just haven't healed yet so you use food or booze as a way to take the edge off. You don't believe you can cope so you use food/booze to bolster you up.

Your weight has weighed you down in life to such a degree that it feels like you're simply existing. You know that opportunities and special moments are passing you by, and you're sitting on the sidelines of your life.

What if being overweight was one of the biggest gifts of your life and you just haven't realized it? Did you roll your eyes? The women at my live events do until I expand on this concept. When you get truly honest with yourself and understand exactly where you are in life: overweight, sedentary, in a life rut, facing illness, or whatever might be going on for you, and you make the decision to take charge of your health, it's the biggest gift you can give yourself. You see, your soul is asking – no, begging – you to wake up and take care of yourself. The messages have been coming to you for years, possibly decades, but you've ignored them, you've taken care of other people instead.

Now, with this weight problem, your heart of hearts self is trying to get your attention and say, "Hey, beautiful, this is not meant to be your life. I need you. I need you to love me and take care of me." Truly, if you've read this far in this book, I want you to understand this, you are being presented with the opportunity of a lifetime. You truly understand that it's not about the pounds you're going to lose, it's about healing from the inside out. It's about learning how to prioritize and love yourself.

Here's what I can tell from having once been in your shoes. Time is going to pass regardless of what you choose to do. But

I can tell you from personal experience and from watching hundreds of other women transform their bodies and their lives, that it takes *way* more emotional energy to stay stuck than it does to change. Both are hard. But the emotional energy that gets expended feeling like a fat failure who hides from the beautiful things in life, choosing not to be seen or fully participate in life is way more painful than expending your emotional energy on learning how to choose you and lose weight and be healthy. Being overweight is a concrete, tangible, visible sign that you are out of emotional alignment with yourself. What you don't change, you choose.

The reason that weight loss is so difficult for women is that it's way deeper than just what foods you eat or how you move your body. I've said it before if all it took was knowledge to lose weight, every woman would effortlessly be a size two. Over five billion results pop up when I search "weight loss" on Google. There's a ton of information out there. You're smart. If I asked you what you thought you needed to do to lose weight you could probably tell me at least five things that would make a huge difference for you. The question is, why don't you do them?

This is why.

Losing weight requires you to go on a Soul Journey where you address the Big 4 which includes the head, heart, body, and soul. It can seem almost impossible, especially if you're at your wit's end with your weight loss but let me show you how Tara, a 45-year-old woman who battled weight loss her whole life, did this when she was exactly where you are now.

Head

One of the things that the popular diet books/programs don't teach you is that getting into the right mindset for weight loss is critical. Perhaps you've heard the saying, "Where your mind goes is where energy flows." If you try to start your weight-loss journey already engaging in self-doubt, convinced that nothing works for you, and feeling hopeless, do you think you have the chance to be successful? No. Because your mindset is creating your expectations. Most women expect to fail at weight loss and then they do. Part of the reason for this is that they simply don't have access to the correct information. The misinformation that exists is mind-blowing and it truly hurts my heart when smart women tell me all of these dumb weight loss myths that they've become a victim to. And yet, I get it.

Tara came to me with a four-year degree in kinesiology and was a registered nurse. Since her early twenties, Tara had tried every diet out there. She lived her twenties and thirties feeling deprived, restricted, and terrorized herself with punishing rules around food and grueling exercise at the gym. Losing weight for her was like a slow form of torture that was robbing her spirit for life. The years of listening to the misinformation in the dieting world had destroyed her ability to think rationally about her body, food, and her weight. Instead she was obsessive, compulsive, and addicted to the quick fix. The diet industry had indoctrinated so much misinformation in Tara she was unable to discern truth from myth in spite of her incredible education.

Tara felt angry, frustrated, and desperate – she was willing to do whatever it took to lose the weight and didn't care how she needed to do it. Diet pills, injections, and even surgery were on her radar. She wanted the weight gone now.

Focusing on your head also means having the appropriate physiological expectations of fat loss for your body. It drives me crazy when women think that they should be able to lose five pounds week after week after week. If that's what you think is successful, then you will always fail because for most, that's a faulty expectation. The wrong information can set you up with false hope. The challenge with this is women don't like how slow true, permanent weight loss is. They get impatient and try to rush the result. It doesn't work.

Tara bumped into an old friend, Sonya, who she hadn't seen for years and who also happened to be a client of mine. Sonya had lost twenty-five pounds and Tara was shocked. She'd never seen her friend looking so happy and healthy. Tara was incredulous. She peppered Sonya with questions wanting to know how she'd created this transformation in her life. Sonya beamed with pride and shared openly about the weight loss program she was doing with me (remember Sonya? She was the woman who came to my live event who was so stressed and worried about her health and her weight). Sonya stressed that the science-based info she was learning in my program plus being part of my private weight loss community were the two things that had contributed to her incredible success. She now knew better so she could do better.

The reason being in a weight-loss community is so important is that you need to surround yourself with other women, just like you, who are learning how to think about weight loss in a whole new way. You have to insulate yourself from the dieting rhetoric and be taught how to think new thoughts so you can feel differently about yourself and end the mean conversation in your head.

Heart

As I talked about in chapters 10 and 11, if you use food to stuff down your feelings instead of feeling them, then weight loss is almost impossible. You have to breathe in courage and exhale fear and trust that you can handle whatever is going on in your life. You need to become willing to heal past hurts and practice the art of letting go. So often, if hard and horrible things have happened, it's easy to hold a grudge or want to blame and stay angry. The only person that energy is hurting is you.

Women work so hard to keep the mask of "fine" on when they're crumbling on the inside.

They pretend that everything is fine when it's not. It's a standard answer to so many questions:

"How are you doing?" – "Fine."

"How's your family?" – "Fine."

"How are things going for you?" – "Fine."

"How's your marriage?" – "Fine."

It's the ultimate cop-out answer and usually there's a big fake smile that goes along with the word.

It's like somehow if you keep "holding it all together" everything will be fine. What a lie. This is a perfect example of how you're lying to yourself because eventually, you're going to break. This may come in the form of divorce, illness, or depression. Maybe it already has.

Tara experienced this in every way. She had just been through a difficult divorce that had left her with nothing. She felt empty inside except for the anger at her ex-husband and the regret for the years she felt she wasted. There was a deep sadness that accompanied her anger and all of it was bundled up inside. She was an expert at using chips and beer to stuff it down. After running into Sonya, Tara went home and binged on something different, my podcast.

After hours of listening, the one thing that sunk in for Tara was that she'd been putting all of her effort on the external things (what she ate, how she worked out, dieting rules, what she wasn't allowed to eat and so forth) and was neglecting what was going on in her heart.

She realized my message was clear. For an outer transformation to happen, you have to do your inner work. It's about getting in touch with your feelings and being able to know what's going on for you. If you're using food or booze to numb the pain, then you are also numbing the joy that you're able to experience in your life. It's not a one-sided analgesic. This is why so many women like Tara feel like they're "blah" and trapped in a life rut.

Tara's life changed forever that night. She reached out, connected with me and began to do the real work. If you know that you have Heart Work to do, be gentle with yourself. Embrace compassion but don't stay complacent. It's time to put pen to paper and pour your heart on to the pages otherwise the pain stays trapped inside.

My favorite way to start doing Heart Work is by doing this exercise first thing in the morning in my journal. It's called Sentence Completion Work; essentially, it's a brain rewiring exercise. You take the beginning of the sentences written below (the sentence stem) and then as quickly as possible you write as many endings as you can in two minutes. The goal is to have a minimum of six full sentences and a maximum of ten. Don't overthink. Don't judge. Don't try to get it "right." Just write. Here's an example of what this looks like:

"If I was kinder to myself..." (sentence stem)

- *Life would feel easier and I wouldn't feel so stressed all the time*
- *I'd make better choices*
- *I would be nicer to my husband*
- *I'd be more joyful and laugh more*
- *I wouldn't beat myself up for making mistakes*
- *My life would be happier*
- *I wouldn't eat as much, I wouldn't need to, I'd like myself more*
- *I'd forgive myself for mistakes in my past*

This forces your brain to think about things in your life in a different way, a way other than what is your habitual thinking. The minute that you allow yourself to create a new thought or to look at something in a new way you've opened up the possibility of creating a new truth to grab on to.

Set a timer for ten minutes and complete this exercise now. If this takes you longer than ten minutes it means that you're getting caught up in perfectionism and thinking of a "good" response, you're already judging yourself. Let your mind open up and just write, take approximately two minutes for each sentence stem.

Sentence Stems (complete six to ten endings for each statement below):

1. If I believed I was truly "enough"...
2. If I truly forgave myself...
3. If I were to express 5 percent more of who I am...
4. If I were to admit what's painful for me to feel...
5. If I loved myself deeply...

Reflect on what you just wrote and then ask yourself this question, "If any of what I wrote is true, it might be helpful if I..." and make some new decisions in your life. This is how you choose to do Heart Work and begin the process of healing.

Body

Your body matters. Every aspect of your body matters. You must learn how to nourish it. How much food does your body need? What does it feel like to overeat? How does your body like to move? It's time to stop being critical of your body and get curious about it instead.

Tara spent over two decades nitpicking her body – everything from her lack of thigh gap to her belly bulge which created the dreaded muffin top over her jeans, as she described it. She punished it, abused it, ridiculed it and hated it and yet longed to love her body and feel at home in it.

Your body is your forever vehicle. It's the only vehicle you have to get through life with. Every single experience you have is conducted through you being in your body. How well are you treating it? Do you expect it to hold up well over time? Compare your body to your car. My hunch is that you have spent way more money, time, and effort on taking care of your car than you have your physical body.

You had to buy your car so you spent money on it, and then you have to maintain your car. That means putting gas into it, getting the oil changed, repairing the breaks and changing the timing belts when necessary. You may love your car, so you take it to a car wash once a week and get it detailed once a month. What if you took just as good of care of your physical body as you do your car? This metaphor resonated loudly with Tara as she drove a Range Rover and took immaculate care of it. She asked herself why she respected a piece of metal more than she respected herself? It was a question that left her in tears.

Tara recognized that she was completely out of alignment with what she wanted to feel like in her body and in how she thought about it and treated it. Perhaps, you can relate? The only way to change how you feel about your body is to change the way you think about it. From there, you get to change what you *do* with your body. And make no mistake, what you do with your body matters. It responds to your efforts. It responds to the food you put in it. It responds to the ways you move it.

What's exciting to me is your body is infinitely moldable, shapeable, and changeable. I've been every kind of "fit" there is from marathon fit to gym fit, to Ironman fit to not fit at all. You get to make a decision about the kind of body you want to live in. Tara decided that she wanted to honor her body and be kind to it. She wanted to step away from the pattern of abuse and harsh workouts she'd previously punished herself with. It was time for her to create peace with her body so yoga became her thing. So did walking. After that felt good she began working out again in the gym but had a different mindset around it and it was fun. Tara is now at home in her body. She feels good in it. She likes how it looks naked (and with clothes on). She's fit and free.

Feeling confident, strong and at home in your physical body is the greatest gift you can give yourself. What I know is that until a woman is truly willing to nourish herself physically, mentally, emotionally, spiritually, and sexually, weight loss will be a struggle. It doesn't have to be. This is where your soul work comes in.

Soul

The final element of the Big 4 is your soul. I believe that we all have soul cravings and when we ignore those they turn into food cravings. A concrete example of this is love. I believe every human being craves love. We need love to feed our souls and to survive. Our deepest fears around not being enough extend to not being enough to be loved. That somehow you're not worthy of that. And that's terrifying. Beyond love, there's emotional intimacy, the ability to know yourself at the most intimate level and to allow others to as well.

The problem with this piece, the soul piece, is the person's love we crave the most is our own. What if you unconditionally loved and accepted yourself the way you do your child or niece? What would be different for you? Instead, you've spent years or decades hating pieces of yourself. Your emotional energy has been spent criticizing the way you look, specific body features, all the things that are wrong with you. You've spent your inner dialogue tearing yourself down instead of building yourself up. No wonder you seek comfort in food.

This was no different for Tara. The years that she spent in a loveless marriage where she believed her needs didn't matter had taken a toll on her essence. She'd forgotten who she was and stopped believing in herself. It was far simpler to focus on her weight issues and spend her energy looking for the next diet. In order to move forward with her weight loss goals, Tara needed to come back to herself and learn how to unconditionally love herself. This may be the toughest job of all.

This is the inner work that most women fail to do. Dieting doesn't teach you this. In fact, dieting propagates your self-hate. I'd like to help you fix this but I'm going to be completely transparent here – this is challenging work and to be honest it's lifelong work – that's why it's called "Soul" work, you're always evolving. But you can start it now, today, by choosing to decide that you matter. You can choose to love yourself instead of hating yourself. You can choose to change.

The fact that you're reading this right now means you're already doing this work. You're getting curious instead of being critical. You're opening yourself up to a new way of doing things. You're choosing to grow and change instead of staying stuck with what isn't working. All of that is Soul Work.

Complex, right? Maybe. Or maybe it's simple. Choose you. Pay attention to what you need and want and allow that to be important. Laugh. Love. Play. Stop taking yourself and life so seriously. And remember the woman you dreamed of being because she's in you now. Going on a weight-loss journey where you get to the roots of the dandelion is what allows you to find her.

Tara started her journey when she was at the lowest place in her life and now, four months later, she's a new woman with a new outlook on life, herself, her health. She disrupted her life by changing her addiction to the dieting industry. If she can, so can you.

When you challenge yourself to get real with who you currently are and the choices you've made in the past and forgive yourself instead of judging yourself – that's when the magic happens. That's when you start to see results that last because you're no longer drowning yourself in food or booze to numb your pain.

Even when you choose to do all of the above, there still can be certain dieting pitfalls that you stumble into. This next chapter is all about what those pitfalls are and how to avoid them so you can stay focused on your vision.

14

The Real Reasons You Stay Stuck

"She slept with the wolves without fear, for the wolves knew a lion was among them."
—R.M. Drake

By now you might be nodding your head with a basket full of tissues beside you because reading this has touched an emotional nerve that rings with truth. And you want it – all of it. You want to release the weight for good, you want greater access to your feelings and to be able to let go of things from the past. You know the strategies and tactics and all of the content makes sense, so what gets in the way and how do you avoid these dieting pitfalls?

Your Habits

You have become accustomed to living life the way you're living it so while you desire to change it can feel like a lot of work to start and so you create excuses. You tell yourself things like this isn't the right time, you don't have the energy to focus on this right now, it's too hard, and that you'll do it later when you're less busy. When I use the word "habits," I'm referring to your habitual thoughts, feelings, and actions. The way you think is a habit.

Women stay stuck and engaged in their losing battle of weight loss for a million reasons. I've already discussed many of these but let's sum them up here.

You Don't Have the Right Knowledge

Your life is busy, and you just don't have the time to research the five billion Google hits for weight loss and sort through the information. Because you don't understand food and metabolism or what's required for fat loss in a science-y way you get lost in the sea of lies and it's easier to just try to follow the diet hype. Except it's not because you never get the lasting results you want.

I started down that path and luckily for me I experienced my "God moment" and was able to choose a different route. You get to do that too. You're almost at the end of this book which means you know better, when you know better you can do better. If you can't see yourself doing what you're doing five years from now then you're on a diet and it's time to stop. It's time for you to trust yourself. If you're doing something that feels icky or unsustainable then it is. If you know you've been letting yourself off the hook, then it's time to recommit to yourself.

If you don't have the time to become a weight loss expert then find someone who is and work with them. It will save you so much frustration and allow you to achieve your goal, for real this time.

You're Impatient

Weight loss is a long-play game. This isn't a thirty-day effort. It's not about being on a program, or a cleanse or detox. It's about creating a lifestyle that you can live with for the rest of your life where you get to have freedom with food. True, lasting weight loss is slow. Slower than you want it to be and you lacked the emotional endurance it takes to stay fully committed because you're tired, and feel alone, and are dealing with all of life's stresses on your own.

Let's change the rules of the game. Pull out your calculator. Write down the amount of weight you want to lose and then divide that number by five. That's how many months it's going to take for you to get to your goal *without* dieting. Now you can have the proper timeframe to base your weight loss success on. Here are examples from my clients who've lost weight and here's how long it took them:

Yvonne: Thirty-five pounds divided by five equals seven months. It took her six months to lose her weight, she's shopping for new clothes now.

Andrea: Twenty pounds divided by five equals four months. Andrea has gained and lost the same twenty or thirty pounds eight times. She always did it quickly with a fad diet. She's currently halfway through my twelve-week program and has lost seven pounds eating *normally*. She's thrilled.

Kim: Forty-seven pounds divided by five equals approximately nine and a half months. It took her ten months to complete her weight-loss journey and she's kept it off for two years.

Megan: Thirty-five pounds divided by five equals seven months. It took Megan nine months as she had a ton of self-sabotaging behaviors that she needed to work through. For the first time in her life, she's comfortable in her body. She trusts it and takes care of it.

There are two ways to approach weight loss – the first is what 99 percent of what most overweight women want and spend most of their lives trying to create and sustain and that's fast weight loss, the weight comes off but doesn't stay off. The second approach is to lose weight in a different kind of way where you know you're not going to regain it. It's slower but you choose to do it this way because the gazillion other ways that you've tried haven't worked. This is slow, steady, healthy, permanent weight loss. This is what I teach.

You might not think that losing five pounds a month is great considering there are plenty of diet programs saying you can lose five pounds a week, but then I trust that you're smart enough to realize that the dieting industry is savvy. They sell women what they want but never, ever give them what they crave.

It's time to cultivate your patience so you can finally be successful at this – you can lose weight one last time, you just need to do it differently than before. Go slow, stay committed and watch the pounds drop off and stay off.

You Lack Accountability to Yourself

You would do anything for a friend, including getting up at 6 a.m. to go for a walk but if it's just you, you'll hit snooze. You've lied to yourself for so long about what you say you're going to do that you no longer trust yourself. You've broken promise after promise to yourself and now you're skeptical of what you commit to. You expect your failure instead of your success and then create situations for yourself that produce this result and allow you to be right. It's a vicious cycle and it's your habit to stay engaged in it.

It's time to break up with your old ways. No more saying one thing and doing another. The best way to stay accountable is to create a vision of yourself and your life that is so exciting you can't help but take action. It's time to get uncomfortable. If you don't choose to change then nothing will change, including your weight.

The easiest way to set up accountability for yourself is:

1. Create a plan for your success. Write out what your goals are for the month, the week and then create daily goals based on that.

2. Find an accountability buddy and create a relationship where you expect each other to keep your commitments. Don't let your buddy indulge your excuses, ask for them to be kind but firm. In fact, I had one of my business coaches hold me accountable by getting me to agree that if I didn't keep my commitment, I'd donate $500 to a charity I didn't actually support or believe in. Trust me – it worked.

3. Create a reward system for yourself and make it non-food based. Use these little rewards as a way to incentivize yourself to keep going even when you don't feel like it. I have daily, weekly, and monthly rewards for myself. The daily and weekly things are little like allowing myself to watch two or three episodes of a show on Netflix at one time, or getting a massage. The big ones are things like a weekend away or a day at my favorite spa.

4. In the beginning, being accountable to yourself will feel like work. It is work. You're changing your habits.

Your Inner Voice is Mean

Oh, lordy, if anyone got inside your head and heard what you said to yourself, they'd faint due to sadness. Even when you do start seeing results that's when your mean voice gets loudest and tells you that "this won't stick... you're not good at this" and then you remind yourself of all of your failures. You start to believe (again) the mean, hurtful words and turn to wine and chocolate to console yourself telling yourself why bother, it's too much work, and you'll probably just fail anyway. The mean voice wins again.

Here's what you need to know about this nasty voice – it will always be there, mine is speaking loudly in the back of my mind right now as I type this and I'm simply tuning it out, I've had *years* of practice in learning how to do so. I don't care what that voice says but I sure used to. That voice has held me back in my life in so many different ways and my guess is the same is true for you. Here are some ways that voice triggered my insecurities, fears, and self-doubt:

- I didn't go to medical school because it told me I wasn't smart enough
- When I was asked out by this handsome man I said "No" because it told me I wasn't pretty enough and he probably wouldn't like me anyway
- I never asked for help because it told me I didn't deserve it
- I didn't believe that I was "worth it" so never asked for a raise at my old job when all of my colleagues did

I spent years believing crap that this voice told me and it caused me to play small, and not go after the things that I truly wanted in my life. I simply don't allow that to happen anymore. (By the way, that voice is telling me to stop writing this paragraph, that it's dumb and that no one is going to read this book anyway so I should just go watch TV. You see? It's mean.)

For you, the goal is the same. The goal is to no longer listen to that mean voice who tries to hold you back in your life. I want you to stop believing the things it says and instead recognize that it's trying to play a sneaky game where you *stop* making these positive changes for yourself. It doesn't like it when you get uncomfortable or do new things. It feels scared. Unsure. Worried that you're going to fail. It wants you to stop before you even start.

The first step is to simply observe what that mean voice is saying to you. That's it. Just notice. Get curious about your thoughts. Observe your thoughts without judging them. If it helps, write them down and then see if they feel true for you. Ask yourself if there's a better thought you could think? If there is, write it down and choose to think that thought. Be committed to thinking for yourself and not letting the nasty, mean voice rule your world.

Fear

If you're not dieting, you don't know who you'd be. If you got thin, healthy, and fit you have no idea what your life would be like and that feels almost paralyzing. Focusing on your weight and justifying the reasons you don't go after things in your life has been the most effective way you know of to distract yourself from the areas of your life that need your attention.

- Once I lose twenty pounds, then I'll go after that promotion I want
- Once I lose thirty pounds, then I'll start dating
- Once I lose twenty-five pounds, then I'll start having sex with my husband again
- Once I lose forty pounds, then I'll put on my bathing suit and go swim with my kids
- Once I lose thirty-five pounds, then I'll start that business I'm dreaming of

See what I mean? Your weight has been your excuse to hide and play small in your life. If that excuse isn't there, then what?

Stop focusing on your fear and start making your happiness a priority. Drop the "*when this... then that...*" thinking and start to live your life today. Get bold. What if today was all you had left? Would you say no to sex and swimming with your kids? I doubt it... you'd be all in hoping to experience every last minute to its fullest. Don't wait to lose weight to live that way. In fact, living that way is going to help you lose weight.

You Truly Don't Know How to Prioritize Yourself or Needs

Your habit of self-neglect, self-abandonment, and self-deprioritizing is so ingrained in you that you can't even tell when you're sabotaging yourself. You just do it because it's normal. This keeps you on the hamster wheel of weight loss with wanting, trying and failing because you can't see yourself. You don't know how to create or maintain healthy boundaries, so you constantly forget about yourself or tell yourself that what you need and want doesn't matter and justify that stinky thinking by telling yourself that something else is more important.

You Want the Easy Way

With everything else that's going on in your life you just want this to be easy. You're desperately afraid of taking on "one more thing" because you're already overwhelmed as it is. The thing that you don't know though is that who you become along the way of your weight-loss journey allows you to handle everything else in your life in a better way too. It's not just your weight that changes, you change. You get stronger. You get confident.

You become emotionally resilient. You handle stress better. You have more fun. The easy way will never give you this because you never get the actual thing you want – for the weight to stay off.

Stop expecting that weight loss should happen fast and easy. It's not like that. If it was, you would have already done it. Weight loss is a process. It takes time, knowledge, dedication and support. You need to be willing to get out of your comfort zone and break free from a dieter's mindset. Instead of wishing for something to be different than it is, accept the truth.

You Do Too Much at Once and Nothing Sticks

I see this over and over again with women. They get super clear that they want to lose weight and decide to do whatever it takes and so they make a list that looks something like this:

- Do five cardio sessions a week
- Strength train three times a week
- Stop drinking alcohol
- Eat completely organic
- Don't go out to eat
- Meditate for an hour every day
- Write in my journal twice a day focusing on gratitude
- Add in five more things.

But, you're still working full time and have the same stresses and life challenges you did before and now you're somehow going to do all of this? And sure, you do for a week, maybe two and then slowly these things peter out and you're not doing any of them anymore and feel like a failure, again. You don't know which high-priority areas to focus on so out of desperation you try to do everything at once, which is way too overwhelming. So you quit. And the weight stays on.

You Don't Have Any Support or Cheerleaders

Without support, you will fail. Period. You need to have a community to celebrate your wins with and to lean into when life gets hard. When your confidence wanes, you need to have women around you who can remind you that you got this. The weight loss research is consistent in showing that women who have the best-sustained weight loss results are in a community. That's why Weight Watchers was so successful at first.

It's the exact reason I have a private Facebook community for all of my clients to be a part of. I know, I know, social media can be a time-suck but when you surround yourself with people who believe in you and support you, even on the days you feel like giving up, you change. It's easier to stay committed. You start to believe in yourself. The other thing about being with a community of women who are creating change in their life, is they're modeling the way. They know the challenges. They know the ups and downs you're going through. They get that your family might be complaining about your new healthy habits and your friends are constantly asking you to drink wine with them. They can hold you accountable and remind you of why you're doing this in the first place.

So, figure out who your cheerleaders are. Make friends with the women at the gym or your colleague who you notice is eating better. Remember that you become like the five people you hang out the most with, so find the women who are already on a mission to get healthy, lose weight, and create happiness in their lives. They'll help you do the same.

You Fall Off the Wagon and Stay There for Months

This is something that I hear all of the time, "Jen, I can be good for a while but then I fall off the wagon… and stay there… until I see a picture of myself and then I have to gather up all of my energy to start again." Let me be clear. The stop/start approach or chasing Mondays (as I call it), is the hardest one of all. It's emotionally exhausting and you lack the consistency to ever generate lasting results so you constantly feel like a failure. Besides, even talking about "being on a wagon" means that there's the possibility of falling off, so fear is always in the background. This is a classic "Diet Mentality."

Instead, I want you to focus on creating a lifestyle for yourself that allows you to nourish yourself. When you create a lifestyle, as opposed to being on diet, there is no wagon to "fall off" of. You're simply living your life. Some days you may slip and make a choice that isn't awesome. That's ok. If you do, simply course correct and remember that you have the next moment to make a better decision. That's it. It can be simple.

When my client Sam truly grasped this concept *everything* changed for her. Sam used to live by strict dieting rules and if she "slipped" she'd feel like such a failure that she'd eat and eat and eat telling herself that since she'd screwed up she might as well just let it all go. She'd continue this way for weeks feeling horrible about herself and engaging in all sorts of nasty talk in her head. Then something would happen and she'd start a new diet.

When Sam and I worked on her mindset and the idea that she could make a poor choice but it didn't have to ruin her day or mean that she was failing, it shifted her way of being. She stopped being so mean to herself. She'd recognize what she had done and why and *learn* from what she did and figure out the cue/trigger or the emotional reward she was seeking. Instead of feeling ashamed she felt proud of herself more often than not because within the next hour or so she'd recommit to her vision and make choices that felt good for her. With this approach, Sam was able to become consistent and she stopped *chasing Mondays*. Weight loss became easy for her week after week.

There are almost one billion overweight women in the world right now and 325 million women are obese. The above challenges are something that every woman faces and they can be overcome. You have the ability to change your weight but to do so you need to create a disruption in your life – you can no longer continue doing the same things you've been doing and expect to create a different result for yourself. I know it's possible for you. I've done it and I've coached almost a thousand women to long-lasting permanent weight loss. It's your turn.

15

It's Your Time

I wrote this book because I wanted to show women that there is a way out, that you don't have to feel like you're stuck living in a world of diet deprivation and restriction or trying to starve yourself thin. It doesn't work. But the dieting culture is pervasive, and I want to flip it on its head and create a far better model around how to get healthy – and that's from the inside out. I find that by the time a woman is in her forties or beyond, she's been through some difficult life events – whether that's divorce, betrayal, heartbreak, career shakedown, infertility, elderly or dying parents, sick children, or financial crisis. There's usually a reason she gained the weight.

You're tired of being fed lies. You're ready to hear the truth and you're ready to deal. But you want clarity and real answers that are based on research, not someone's desire to make a quick dime off of a protein shake. It's why you're now at the end of this book.

I get that weight loss can feel crazy-making. It's costing you your energy, sanity, self-confidence, and happiness. At the beginning of this book, it was incredibly important to me that you knew you were in the right place and not alone in your struggle. There are other women who have had the same struggles and desires as you. After coaching hundreds of women, I know how easy it is to think weight loss is so easy for everyone else and somehow you're the problem child. Not true. The struggle can feel real and there is a way out.

Being able to share my God moment with you in chapter 2 is a privilege. For so long, I felt humiliated and embarrassed that I let myself get to that desperate point in my life because I felt like such a failure. And I was scared that I would be judged. I mean, here I am with two university degrees, was a personal trainer and multi-marathoner yet I was carrying so much extra weight. Now I take solace in modeling the fact that knowledge isn't enough and simple diet formulas don't work. It's putting the pieces of that knowledge together in the right way and then doing the deeper emotional work that will allow you to lose the weight for good.

If you can't tell by now, I loathe the diet industry. Yet I'm a part of it. My goal is to use the power of my voice and the written word to do *good* in this industry and to disrupt it. Women deserve to know the truth about what true, lasting weight loss requires and that there is a right way to do it and a wrong way. Most of the dieting industry is built upon fad superficial tactics, weight loss supplements, or convincing you that you need to exercise more, none of which are sustainable for the long-term. The cycle of disappointment and failure this creates for a woman is heartbreaking and needs to stop. Hopefully, by the time you finished reading chapter 3, your hope has been restored and you now believe you can do this. The only thing your past dieting failures mean, is that you now know what doesn't work for you!

Having access to the right information is powerful and when you take a look at how the weight-loss deck is stacked against you, as chapter 4 illustrated, I hope you now realize that you have to be your own ally and advocate. The food industry can't be trusted and if you continue thinking you don't need to dig up the roots of your dandelion then permanent weight loss will be a dream. Understanding that you're a kitty cat living in a lion-sized world can change everything for you. It can de-personalize the challenge of weight loss, allow you to stop blaming your body, or what you considered a "broken or bad" metabolism and now know that you get to create the results you want.

Chapter 5 went deep into making sure you truly get how physiologically and psychologically damaging dieting is and my goal is that no matter what you choose to do tomorrow, you'll never, ever be seduced by a fad diet again. If that's the least of what happens, I'd consider that a huge win. Once you discover the real reason you're overweight, which is due to the fact you overeat, you have power. You get to start asking the right questions so you can come up with better solutions.

In chapter 6, my whole goal was to help you gain awareness around the self-sabotage phenomenon. Understanding the Cycle of Change can set your free because you now have a framework for what you go through and you'll be able to spot fear a mile out or at the very least you can expect a surprise attack. Thank goodness because before, fear stopped you in your tracks.

Charles Duhigg is a genius. He presented habit creation and change in such a simple way and it had a profound effect on my life. The purpose of chapter 7 was to help you gain insight into your habits and for you to recognize what drives your behavior with food. It's not *just* about wanting the chocolate or the wine, it's about the deeper emotional nourishment that you're craving but not getting so you're swapping in a cheap, convenient substitute. Whoa... it's hard-hitting, isn't? But when you get that after years of feeling out of control with food, and you realize you get to be 100 percent in control of your thoughts which drives your feelings and creates your actions which generate your outcomes – did you have the light bulb moment when you realized *you* have had all the power all along? You just didn't know it.

Ideal weight loss results are a combination of doing the right things in the right order. Actions are important, but you need to take the right, committed actions, not half-assed ones that generate a mediocre result. When you set your environment up to support the habits, you're trying to change you're giving yourself a huge advantage and chance to win the weight loss battle. Chapter 8 explained why relying on willpower and discipline is futile, they're like muscles that fatigue over time. This is a huge relief, don't you think? No longer can you blame your lack of willpower for your inability to lose weight; it's not about that. It's about implementing simple tweaks in your lifestyle and truly understanding how to create a weight loss result that lasts.

I hope you now get that exercise isn't the answer to your weight loss struggles. As a clinical exercise physiologist and weight loss expert, you get to trust me on this one. I've done the research and know that using exercise as a weight-loss tool will cause you to fail every time. Chapter 9 explained this thoroughly. You need to nourish yourself physically and that does mean moving your body. There are a gazillion health benefits you get from being regularly active. Being sedentary is the enemy of health. I believe that knowing that even ten minutes of gentle exercise can make a difference is positive and uplifting, don't you?

The weight loss, nutrition, and health world has become so confusing. There's misinformation, fear, doubt, skepticism, and a general lack of trust out there which makes it hard to get traction and create results for yourself. What I've witnessed over and over again is how important it is to go back to the weight loss basics. Are you taking good care of yourself? Are you getting good sleep, eating real (non-processed food), and handling your stress well? Chapter 10 is critical for helping you identify the other key lifestyle components that are essential for weight loss to happen. Skip these and kiss permanent weight loss goodbye.

I've probably said it at least half a dozen times that if weight loss was easy, every woman would be a size two. Don't get me wrong, weight loss is *simple* – there are certain factual things based in body science that if you were to do them with consistency, you'd lose weight. Why don't you? Because it's not *easy*. You are an emotional, social being who has a range of human emotions that you deal with every single day of your life and that's what makes weight loss complicated. When you get crystal clear with yourself and truly understand that to lose weight for the last time, you've got to deal with healing the relationship you have with yourself, you're truly 80 percent of the way there. Promise. Chapter 13 presents the Big 4 and the beauty of attending to these often-neglected areas.

It would be neglectful of me as a weight loss expert if I didn't tell you the real-life challenges that you are going to face, or that you have possibly already encountered on your weight-loss journey. Knowledge is power. When you personalize these challenges and think that you're the only woman who experiences them, you dump boatloads of shame onto yourself and you already have enough of that. All women encounter these barriers or roadblocks, it's how you choose to blast through them that matters. Expect them and trust you can handle it. Now that you know what might get in your way, you can get proactive instead of reactive and quitting. When you know better, you can do better. It's that simple.

Finally, my true reason for writing this book is that the world needs women right now more than it ever has before in the history of time. This world needs women who are willing to stand up and speak up about what's not right, women who are strong and willing to take action. All you need to do is turn on the TV, or read the news, it's depressing. The world needs women leaders, women's voices, and have the benefit of women's contribution to the global conversation on equality, health, education and so on.

Here's what I know about being an overweight woman, it takes a toll on your confidence. You start to shrink back, get quiet and have a desire to not be seen – you don't want attention to be drawn to you. You want to be invisible. And I'm begging for you to stop. It hurts you, your family, your community and our world. I believe in you. I know what's possible for you when you inhale courage and exhale fear. But there are no shortcuts. Dieting is a shortcut and life just doesn't work that way. You've got to do the real work, it's 100 percent worth it.

I want women around the world to feel free, find their confidence, tap into their intuitive wisdom, their passion and creativity, their deepest desires and have the confidence to go after whatever it is they want in life. I want women to believe that they are *enough*. I want *you* to believe that you are *enough*. I want you to know that you are enough exactly as you are and that you value does *not* come from being a size two but by who you are.

Women's voices are powerful. When your weight is holding you back in life it's holding you back from accessing the whole experience of your life – everything from your sense of self, to the emotional and physical intimacy you create for yourself, to your career choices, the relationships you have with your spouse, family, kids, and friends – even your bank account. Trust me, there is never a good time to lose weight or to learn how to prioritize yourself. The best time is right now.

I believe in women. I know that women overestimate what they can do in a month and underestimate what they can do in a year. If I've reignited your hope and inner resolve to go after your weight loss goal *one* more time but you'll do it differently, then I got to make a difference. Shift your thinking, shift your mindset, and dramatically shift the results you create.

It's time to disrupt the diet industry.

Acknowledgments

This book has been in my heart for years now and it's a dream come true to actually have completed it. Writing a book is not a solitary endeavor and there are so many people in my life who supported and loved me in incredible ways during this process. It's a privilege to honor you all.

Ley, you are the love of my life and I can't thank you enough for the cups of coffee you brought me, the dinners you made, and times you listened to me rattle around my countless ideas as I tried to create sense in my head of what I wanted this book to be about. Not to mention all of the late night snuggles as I climbed into bed after a long night of typing. It's through you that I know what unconditional love is. You are my everything – forever and always.

Jake and Liv, my little loves, you two have been the best at encouraging me. Liv, I'll never forget when you got home from school, came into the office, hugged me, and said, "Run towards your dreams, Mama." I have, and I will continue to do so. And Jake, you asked me so many great questions about my book and the writing process. When I was stuck, you always knew the right thing to say to help me and make me laugh. You are such incredible children. Both of you are wise beyond your years and have the biggest hearts. The best gift I've ever received are you two and what I love most is watching you two chase your own dreams.

I'm blessed with angels who seem to drop into my life to accompany me on this crazy entrepreneurial journey of mine. Emily, you were the first. Your willingness to believe in me and go through the ups and downs as I learned along the way meant the world. I know working with me can be like riding a roller coaster – lots of twists and turns, but the ride is adventurous and fun and we get to create profound impact together in this world. You keep things operating smoothly, never losing your cool and running the team like a rock star. Thank you.

Melonie, you are an angel here on earth. From the minute we met, your unwavering faith and belief in me, my message, and the Diet Disruption Movement has been incredible. Your honesty, humour, and wisdom are true gifts that I've been blessed to experience. With you as Magpie and me as Squirrel, we make an incredible team.

This book literally would not have come forth if it wasn't for Angela Lauria, CEO and founder of the Author Incubator. Within the first five minutes of hearing you speak about the difference writing a book could make in the world, I knew I'd found my writing mentor. To my developmental editor, Mehrina Asif, my editor, Nkechi Jennifer Obi, and my managing editor, Cory Hott, thank you for making this process so incredibly seamless and for providing me with endless support. Your encouragement and belief in my message kept me going. There are many more people at The Author Incubator who deserve thanks – know you are in my heart.

To my amazing clients! It is through you that this book became possible. Each and every one of you have been extraordinary to work with. It is a privilege and an honor that you chose me to help you create disruption in your life so that you could shed the emotional and physical weight that was holding you back. I'm in awe of all of you. This work requires you to be brave and bold; vulnerable and committed; fierce and passionate. I will forever hold you in my heart and give thanks to the lessons you taught me. Go give your gifts to the world.

Lastly, Mom – I love how proud you are of me and how you are always in my corner. Thank you for teaching me how to be resilient in life. I love you dearly.

Thank You

Reading a book from cover to cover is a huge accomplishment. Thank you for taking the time to go through these pages. It tells me that you are well on your way to creating lasting weight loss success in your life. My heart of heart's desire is that you're able to now see things differently and know more about what to do and not do to free yourself from dieting forever.

I'm building my community of incredible women, just like you, one woman at a time and would love to stay connected. Isolation is the enemy of health, happiness, and weight loss. I believe we all do better when we surround ourselves with good women. The easiest way to do that is to join my private Facebook group, Diet Disruption Movement:

http://facebook.com/groups/DietDisruptionMovement

Lastly, if you'd like to grab the accompanying bonuses that go along with this book please go to this website: www.dietdisruptionbook.com/bonuses

With hugs and gratitude,

Jennifer

About the Author

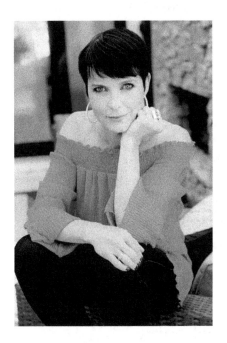

Weight loss expert Jennifer Powter, MSc, could train Olympic athletes if she wanted to. Happily for us, she doesn't. Instead, Jennifer coaches successful women with imperfect lives who want to finally break free from dieting and lose the weight for good this time.

The $70 million dieting industry preys on the insecurities of women – and as the Diet Disruptor, Jennifer is taking a stand.

Her revolutionary approach to weight loss goes against the traditional grain, demolishing the dieting myths that have held women hostage for so long.

As well as holding a master's degree, Jennifer is a qualified clinical exercise physiologist, a double-certified health and life coach, and an emotional intelligence practitioner. She has also experienced her own transformational weight loss journey, permanently losing more than thirty-five pounds that had held her back from living her best life.

Over the last twenty years Jennifer has helped thousands of women reclaim their bodies and minds, using her unique, soulful approach and proven Metabolic Profile Index (MPI) assessment to help every woman determine exactly what she needs, emotionally and metabolically. She breaks down the science of physiological transformation into six simple and empowering steps – so healthy weight loss becomes a joy.

Jennifer is one of the nation's leading health experts, a sought-after speaker, and creator of the Diet Disruption Podcast. She lives near the breathtaking Rocky Mountains in Calgary, Alberta, with her family and their gorgeous St. Bernard, Harley.

CPSIA information can be obtained
at www.ICGtesting.com
Printed in the USA
JSHW021342171220
10332JS00012B/3